Sugar Detox

How to Overcome Sugar Addiction NOW

and for the Rest of Your Life

Charlotte Young

ISBN-13: 9781630220839

Table of Contents

Publishers Notes

Disclaimer

This publication is intended to provide helpful and informative material. It is not intended to diagnose, treat, cure, or prevent any health problem or condition, nor is intended to replace the advice of a physician. No action should be taken solely on the contents of this book. Always consult your physician or qualified health-care professional on any matters regarding your health and before adopting any suggestions in this book or drawing inferences from it.

The author and publisher specifically disclaim all responsibility for any liability, loss or risk, personal or otherwise, which is incurred as a consequence, directly or indirectly, from the use or application of any contents of this book.

Any and all product names referenced within this book are the trademarks of their respective owners. None of these owners have sponsored, authorized, endorsed, or approved this book.

Always read all information provided by the manufacturers' product labels before using their products. The author and publisher are not responsible for claims made by manufacturers.

If you would like to contact the author, please send an email to Authors@TenFingersPublishing.com

Paperback Edition © 2013

Manufactured in the United States of America

Dedication

This book is lovingly dedicated to all my readers

who are looking to improve their lives through better health.

Believe me when I say, "You can do it!" because I did!

Introduction

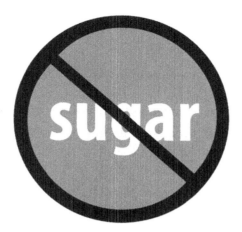

So, you are thinking of doing a sugar detox? Well, congratulations! You are about to embark on an entirely new adventure—one that can result in some stressful moments, yet one where you most likely will discover things about yourself you never realized. Yes, a sugar detox can be quite a learning experience.

As you read this guide, I will share with you much of what you can expect to experience during a sugar detox program—no matter which one you participate in—and there are many. As far as a sugar detox is concerned, many revolve around a certain length of time. I have seen some that challenge you to go 30 days without any sugar—something I have personally done myself. Others are slightly shorter—clocking in at 21 days, a week, 3 days and even 1!

While the length of time varies from program to program, there are many similarities between them. There are certain symptoms you will want to be aware of that many people experience when they withdraw from sugar. There are certain foods you will be asked to avoid for the specified time, and there are tips and sometimes recipes given to help you as you come out of their program.

Realize that no matter which program you choose and how long you plan to eliminate sugar from your diet, any effort you make to eat healthier will benefit you.

In this guide I will share with you:

- How to know if you are addicted to sugar

- How to prepare before you conduct a sugar detox

- Which foods to avoid

- Which foods to consume in larger quantities

- A handy grocery list you can download, print out and take with you to the store

- What to expect as you detox

- How to eat out in restaurants

- And some thoughts on how to make positive changes for the rest of your life

- Plus, as an added bonus, I have some wonderful recipes you can download, print out and use for yourself and your family to help you continue eating healthier without added and hidden sugars in your diet

Now come along with me as I take you by the hand and walk you through a sugar detox each step of the way. By doing so, you will feel empowered and educated about what to expect, and how to succeed with a sugar detox that can ultimately change your health and your life in incredible ways.

Okay. Let's get started!

Chapter 1- How Can I Know If I Am Addicted to Sugar?

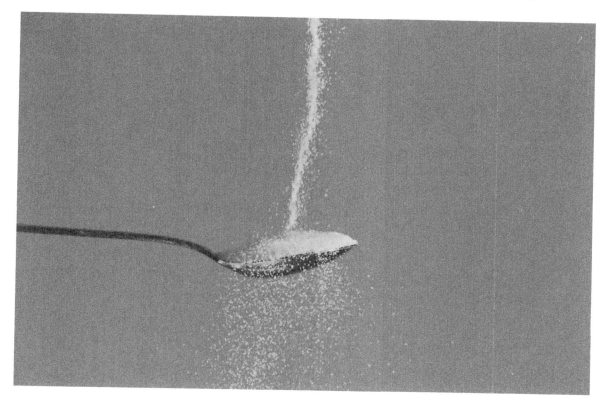

As a kid, I never realized that sugar was something many now consider "addictive." I just remember how much I enjoyed ice cream, lollipops, and a tasty chocolate candy bar. While I still do like these foods, I have dramatically limited my intake of these foods because now I am aware of the kinds of sugar used to prepare them. (Sometimes being a grownup is not as much fun.)

Before we go much farther into this book, you may be asking yourself if this book is for you. I suspect you may very well have a problem with sugar (like I did) because you were curious about the title and wondered if this might be an issue for you. Yet, I congratulate you for wanting to educate yourself about sugar, to discover how it affects your body, where it hides, and how to reduce your intake of it in your diet.

To help satisfy your curiosity, let us begin with a simple test—a test where you can see what you know about sugar and whether or not it is something you have trouble controlling in your diet.

Now, do not worry! It is not a hard test, but it does require you being honest with yourself. You see, in order to decide if a sugar detox is right for you, you have to know what you are dealing with. For many, sugar is something they enjoy on occasion; for others, it has the potential to become their worst nightmare.

Therefore, if you want to learn more of what sugar is, the different names for it, where it can hide, and how you can eliminate or cut back on your consumption of it, then keep reading. You and I are going to walk through this issue together so you will have a better understanding of what sugar addiction looks like.

My plan is not to bore you with too many medical data while supplying you with helpful information to know what this area of life means. Knowledge is power, and it will enable you to affect change in your life for the better. Like me, I think you will discover that this topic is too important to ignore, so I will give you practical and helpful advice for detoxing and supply you with the tools to gain control over sugar so it does not take control over you.

A Simple Sugar Addiction Test

In the quiz I have created below, simply answer "yes" or "no" as honestly as you can to each question. As you answer, keep track of how many "yes" answers you give because these will be used to tabulate your score on the next page. Remember now: Be honest because cheating is not going to help you at all.

A Simple Sugar Addiction Quiz

Answer each question below with a YES or NO	Yes	No
1. Do you ever find yourself eating so much sugar that you actually end up feeling sick?		
2. Have you ever tried to quit eating sugar for a period of time, only to discover that you just could not do it?		
3. Do you consume sugar on a daily basis?		
4. Do you have a difficult time resisting desserts?		
5. Do you have a secret stash of sweets hidden away that others do not know about – so they do not see you when you eat them?		
6. Do you feel fatigued more than you think you should?		
7. Do you often indulge in eating something with sugar because you believe it will make you feel better, only to realize that you feel worse?		
8. After you have eaten a lot of sugar, do you feel guilty, mad at yourself, or even ashamed?		
9. Do you ever "pig out" on sugar because you have told yourself, "This is the last time I am ever going to do this," only to do it again?		
10. Do you ever feel like sugar is "calling your name," and you have to obey?		
11. Is it difficult for you to enjoy just a small amount of sugar—like two mini cupcakes or cookies instead of five or six?		
12. Do you feel like sugar destroys any willpower you possess? Like it somehow is making you overeat and lose control?		
13. Can you honestly have sweets in the house without feeling as though you have to eat them?		
14. Do you think you could stop eating something sweet after only one bite?		

Before going to the next page, be sure you have kept track of the number of "yes" answers you gave.

So, how did you do? Do you think you and sugar have a friendly relationship with each other or do you suspect it may have a hold on you?

Well, here are some guidelines to think about concerning the results of your quiz. While there are certainly other factors that truly determine whether someone is addicted to sugar, these results give you a pretty good idea of where you stand.

Count your "yes" answers and use the following scale to see how you did:

1. 0 – 3 means you do not have much to worry about. It sounds as though you have a good handle on how to control your intake of sugar.

2. 4 – 6 means you need to be on the lookout because sugar may be or could become a problem for you

3. If you had 7 or more "yes" answers, then I am afraid you are most likely addicted to sugar

To think you might be "addicted" to sugar may not seem like a very big deal, but let me help you understand how sugar can affect you in your daily life. Basically, I think it would help to look briefly at the four different stages of any kind of substance addiction—sugar being one of them. In fact, some researchers and nutritional experts have stated that sugar can affect our brains in some of the same ways that cocaine does. What this means, then, is that certain levels of sugar can cause our brains to behave in similar ways as someone who is addicted to cocaine!

Now, let me walk you through the four different stages of what an addiction to sugar could look like but in order for this to be successful, you have to pretend as if you have never had sugar before. I know this may be almost impossible to imagine, but try it and let's see how it goes.

1. Stage One ~ This stage involves experimentation. Let's pretend you are enjoying being with a group of friends walking through a shopping center. Someone spots a big picture window and behind the glass are some beautiful pastries. The smells invite you in and you ask the owner what they are. In disbelief, he states they are pastries, topped with delicious sugary icings. Now, you have heard about "sugar" before, but you have never tried it, so at the urging of your friends and the baker, you buy one and give it a try--just to see if you like it.

2. Stage Two ~ This is the stage when misusing sugar begins. After you finished off that pastry, you discovered you really liked it! In fact, you found that later on that day, you wanted more. In the days and weeks that followed, you made numerous trips to the bakery, each time trying new treats—just to see if you liked them. You discovered that when you ate one, you felt better somehow. You could not really explain it—it just happened. Then you discovered that sugar was in treats like cake, candy, and even drinks. As you found yourself consuming more of the sweet stuff, you sensed something was not quite right. You would tell yourself you needed to wait and eat it in moderation. You would make those decisions in your mind and tell yourself when those times would be, but somehow you always seemed to give in and eat a candy bar, a piece of cake, or a cookie when you told yourself you "shouldn't."

3. Stage Three ~ Abuse of sugar is now a part of your life. You have now reached a point where you feel like you cannot function without your morning cup of coffee loaded with fancy creamers and sugar. The other day you wanted to stop at the bakery like you have been doing a lot lately, but time would not allow you to. You didn't sleep well at all the night before and that late-night snack of ice cream with fudge topping made you feel better momentarily, but it didn't help you get to sleep like you were hoping. Now you are praying the morning passes quickly so you can get to the restaurant downstairs and enjoy that pizza you have been dreaming about and some cookies to go with your soda, too.

4. Stage Four ~ Dependency. Lately you have found yourself wondering why you feel so cranky and irritable. You find your energy level just is not what it used to be and you have started noticing how sluggish you get in between breakfast and lunch, lunch and dinner, dinner and bedtime—things that never used to happen. Curiously, your clothes are tighter than they have ever been. And, so much for being healthy like you used to be. Now it seems like you pick up every cold germ that makes it way into the workplace. You never used to have to take a sick day. What are you supposed to do? How can you go back to life as it used to be? Who can help you?

Can you see yourself in any of these stages? Oftentimes, it is not until we begin to experience symptoms such as irritability, weight gain, crankiness, and problems with sleeping that we begin to consider something is wrong and we need to make some healthy changes. Fortunately, changing our eating habits to include healthier foods is positive and can have some dramatic effects in our health.

As you went through the 14 questions in the sugar addiction quiz, did you sense that you lack willpower—that if you would just decide not to eat sugar, that it should be that simple? Yet, you know that just does not seem to work. Chances are you have tried that before—like, who hasn't? I certainly know that I have felt defeated in the past because I thought if I just had more willpower I would succeed.

Since then, I have learned there is more to willpower than just making up your mind to not eat sugar. Success in avoiding sugar also involves learning how to balance your blood sugar levels because these affect our thinking and moods. This means you have to know what types of foods to eat and understanding how they affect you. The foods we eat eventually affect our intestinal system. Many who are gluten sensitive can tell you how much they suffer when they eat grains and other foods that have gluten in them. While I am sure you know some of this, realize that the foods you eat will definitely affect the chemical balances in your brain, which in turn affect your moods and thinking. When you accept the scientific findings that sugar has a similar effect on your brain as a powerful drug, you can see why we need to take our consumption of sugar seriously.

While there are many similarities between how each of our bodies work, everyone's body is different. A food that affects me may not bother you at all, and vice versa. Some of my friends have real problems with the lactose in dairy products; however, I know for certain this is not an issue for me. I have conducted my own 30-day detox from dairy, and at the end of that time, I slowly reintroduced it into my system. As I did so, I have not had a single symptom show up in my body that usually occurs in people who have lactose intolerance.

So, as we discuss what is involved in a sugar detox, consider talking to your healthcare professional if you decide to do this for yourself. If you happen to eat a lot of sugar and then decide to eliminate it for a time, there may be some complicated issues your body has to deal with that may require some help and intervention from a qualified medical professional.

With that said, let me now take you through the process of understanding what sugar is, how it affects your body, and what you can do about it. Remember, knowledge is power, and with it, you can make changes!

Here's to your success!

Chapter 2 - What Is Sugar?

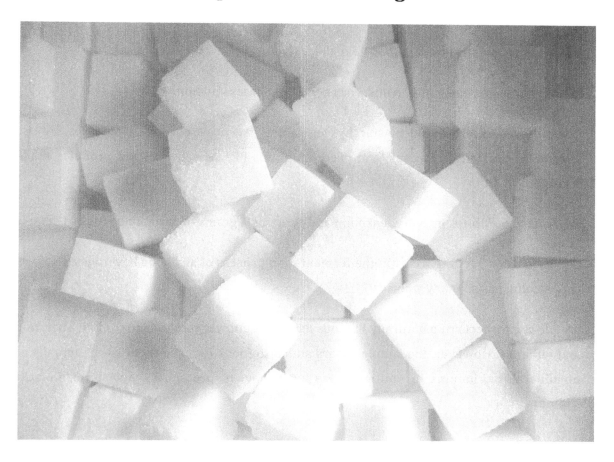

What is sugar? Why, sugar is something that is not hard to find. In fact, you can find it almost everywhere and almost in everything we eat and drink. As you will see later on, sugar can be easily identified in some foods while being sneaky and using an alias to hide in others.

To make this section one you can easily read, I have made a list of some facts about sugar. This will make is easy for you to process the different characteristics of sugar.

1. Sugars are carbohydrates, one of the three main categories of food (proteins, fats, and carbohydrates). Carbohydrates are extremely important for maintaining our health and actually provide our bodies with a source of energy. All foods that are carbohydrates (from table sugar to whole grain bread to broccoli) are broken down by our digestive system to simple sugars as they are ingested into our body.

2. There are several forms of sugar you will recognize: honey, maple syrup, white sugar, brown sugar, raw sugar, cane sugar, corn syrup, high fructose corn syrup, and many others. I will share some of the "scientific" names for sugar later on so you will know how to spot them when you are shopping for your food, eating out, etc.

3. Sugar is a substance that comes from plants like the sugar beet and sugar cane, consisting mostly of sucrose.

4. Sugars are naturally found in foods like dairy (lactose) and fruits (fructose).

5. Simple sugars are present in fruits, corn syrup, molasses and honey.

6. Complex sugars are found in starchy vegetables like peas, corn, and potatoes; non-starchy vegetables like lettuce, greens, and broccoli; grains like wheat, rice, and products made with them.

7. Sugar has 16 calories in every teaspoon and contains 4 grams of carbohydrate per teaspoon.

8. It is used as an agent to assist in the fermentation process of alcoholic beverages. (Now you see why alcohol has so many calories!)

9. Simple sugars occurring naturally in foods like fruits and vegetables also contain fiber, minerals, and vitamins. However, the simple sugars added to foods to make them sweet actually contain no minerals or vitamins. In addition, these sugars have no protein, no cholesterol, no fat, and no sodium.

10. According to the American Heart Association, Americans average about 22 teaspoons of sugar every day! That is 352 calories every day, 2,464 calories a week, and 128,128 calories a year! That is equal to consuming enough calories to gain **1 POUND EVERY 10 DAYS!** While this statistic does not really tell you what sugar is, it may help to explain why we are having trouble losing weight.

11. When we eat something that has a lot of sugar in it, our body ingests it rapidly. However, this causes a spike in the sugar levels of your blood, and in turn, a spike in insulin levels The additional insulin causes the sugar level to drop dramatically, resulting in hunger and cravings for more sugar.

12. Sugar is usually added to foods to provide sweetness and to maintain their quality and freshness.

13. When sugar is added to fruits and vegetables to make jellies and jams, it acts as a preservative.

14. "Sugar" is also a term of endearment (okay, this one does not count but I could not resist!)

As this list indicates, sugar is an important source of energy. It provides nourishment to our bodies and the major energy source in most diets. However, as we will see later on, it can also be a real problem when consumed excessively.

In the next section, I am going to share some of what can happen to your body when you eat too much of this carbohydrate. While there are some symptoms you could probably name right now, there are others that occur inside your body that you may not have realized are happening—that is, until they make themselves known in unpleasant ways.

Let's continue.

Chapter 3 - How Can I Know If I Eat Too Much Sugar?

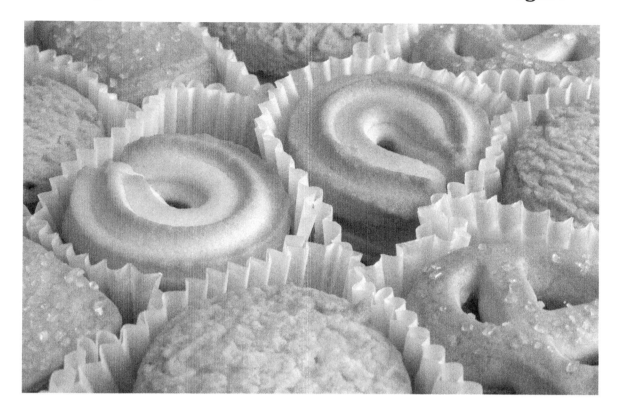

Let us look for a moment at a list of symptoms that can result from having too much sugar in your diet. While this book is certainly not a medical journal, I want you to be aware of some issues and problems you may have experienced or could experience in the future if your sugar consumption is excessive. If, while reading, you discover you are experiencing some of the symptoms listed below, you may decide to examine your intake of sugar and proceed with a sugar detox program.

With some further study, you may find that many symptoms can be alleviated and even reversed when eliminating or cutting back dramatically on your consumption of sugar in your diet. Also, consider talking with your healthcare professional as you learn more information on this topic and how to safely proceed.

Now, take a moment to see if you have any problems or have experienced any of these symptoms that are directly related to eating sugar:

- Cavities

- Diabetes

- Craving carbs

- Allergies

- Gluten Sensitivity

- Headaches

- Bloating

- Overeating—feeling as though you lack willpower

- Difficulty with sleep

- Mood swings

- Fatigue, even to the point of exhaustion

- Feeling anxious

- Being overweight

- Feeling irritable and cranky

- High blood pressure

- Low sex drive

- Problems with feeling depressed

- Acne

- Arthritic inflammation

And, I have to tell you that these are certainly not all of the problems associated with sugar. There are others, but I think you get the idea. Eating excessive amounts of sugar (and I mean eating more sugar than your body needs) does have consequences.

For a moment, let us examine some types of behavior people may exhibit when sugar is a problem in their diet. These symptoms are the result of the ways high levels of sugar affects your brain. In very simple terms, these elevated levels inhibit the production in our brains of its pleasure-producing chemicals like endorphins (natural pain killers), dopamine (helps us think clearly and is a natural energizer), and GABA (our own built-in sedative). Because of its impact on our brain's chemical balance, we will be affected in ways that influence our moods, our ability to think, and even our perception of pain.

Consider for a moment some behaviors you may exhibit or have thought of doing that you did not even realize were related to sugar:

- Have you ever noticed that when you feel stressed, bored, or lonely, you reach for something sugary to eat to help lift your spirits? That is sugar affecting your mood.

- You have secretly hidden a stash of sugary treats that others do not know about (because you do not plan to share with them?) That is sugar affecting your thinking.

- Even though you know that sugary treats are bad for you, have you planned to eat them anyway? That is sugar affecting your thinking.

- Whenever you binge on sweets, do you promise yourself that this is the last time you will ever do it, but secretly you know this is a promise to yourself you cannot keep? Again, that is sugar affecting your thinking.

In Dr. Jacob Teitelbaum's book *Beat Sugar Addiction Now!*, he writes about four different kinds of sugar addicts. (Published by Fair Winds Press, 2010, ISBN-13: 978-1592334155) In brief, they consist of the following groups of people:

- Those who experience cravings resulting from hormone fluctuations like periods and midlife changes such as andropause and menopause

- People with depleted adrenal glands will exhibit irritability and stress when they are hungry

- There are others who rely on sugar and products containing caffeine to "jumpstart" their system. This is usually a sign that they are not getting enough sleep and their nutritional needs should be addressed

- Still others have health issues that worsen with the consumption of sugar such as too much candida (yeast) in their body. Some symptoms tend to be recurrent sinus congestion and infections, symptoms of irritable bowel syndrome, and even spastic colon

As you can see, sugar can cause some complicated side effects in our bodies that influence how we think and feel—something I never would have guessed as a kid.

In the next chapter, I will offer a simple explanation of how sugar can become an addiction.

Chapter 4 – How Can Sugar Be Addicting?

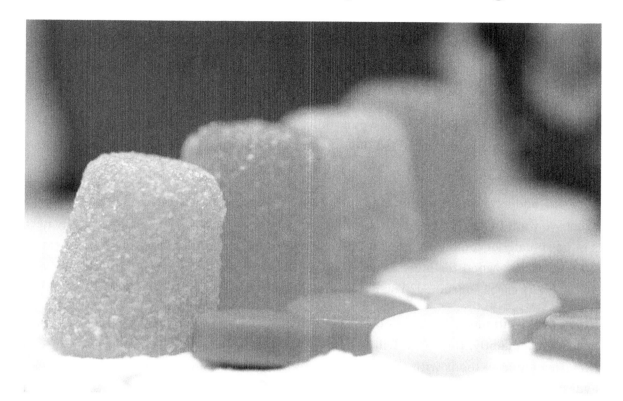

Our bodies are truly incredible machines and one of the things they do is try to maintain a constant level of glucose running through our blood stream. Despite our best efforts to bombard our bodies with an excess load of sugar on occasion, our bodies work hard to keep the sugar level in our bloodstream in check.

For instance, let me show you the process of what happens when you eat a meal that has a high level of sugar in it (I promise to keep it simple.)

- Let's say you have just finished enjoying a meal or snack that had a lot of carbohydrates in it.

- In response, your blood signals your pancreas that there is a new load of sugar running through your system and it needs to shoot out a bunch of insulin into your blood stream so the glucose can be taken into your cells to bring the glucose levels down—and do it in a hurry

- The problem is you shoved in a lot of sugar into your body in a short amount of time, so your system had to react quickly to bring things back down to normal; ironically, in doing so, the end result created a drop in your blood sugar. Oops! Out of balance to be sure

- When this happened, the heavy hit of insulin caused your blood sugar levels to go down below the normal one teaspoon of glucose in your bloodstream, so do you know what this means?

- It means you suddenly became hungry, irritable, and even shaky. Now, do you know what your body wants you to do?

- It wants you to feed it...again...after you just ate not so long ago!

The entire process is actually more complicated than this because sugar also causes the release of serotonin--something many refer to as the "feel good hormone." Serotonin is a hormone that affects areas of your life such as your behavior, your ability to sleep, and your desire to eat. When serotonin levels are high, you usually feel great and life is good; when they are low, you can become irritable and tiredness sets in.

Because our bodies crave serotonin, and serotonin levels are increased by a high carbohydrate diet, guess what we want to eat? The problem is, we often eat more carbohydrates than we really need. This results in us actually becoming somewhat desensitized to the amount of serotonin, so we eat more in order to receive the "good feelings" associated with higher serotonin levels. Can you figure out the result of too many carbs consumed? You got it - weight gain!

This cycle will continue as long as you eat foods that are high in their sugar content and are loaded with carbs. Consequently, this cycle will never be changed or amended until you learn to eliminate empty calories found in foods with added sugars and begin to eat more of the foods that are lower in carbohydrates.

While we are on the subject of eating foods with too many carbs, here is something else you may not be aware of. Because all carbohydrates are made up of sugars, foods like bread, pasta, bagels, and other wheat-laden foods are converted to sugar in your body after you eat them! Bummer huh? This is one of the places where sugar hides in your food. What this means is, it is not only sugar as we know it that causes blood sugar spikes in your body. Your blood sugar levels spike every time you eat the crust of your favorite pizza, the pasta you love under your spaghetti sauce, and the bagel you feast on for breakfast.

I hope it is beginning to become clearer to you that eating too many carbs will result in making you fat. As long as you continue to eat foods high in carbohydrates, like...

- Sugar

- Whole grains

- Refined flours

- Non-fat dairy products because the fats normally a part of a dairy product actually slows down blood sugar spikes. Remove the fat and lactose (sugar in dairy) dominates.

- Low-fat foods, because sugar is usually added when the fats are removed

...The cycle of wanting to feel better about yourself, but finding yourself wanting to eat too many carbs, is only going to continue until you make changes in the kind of foods you eat.

To help you begin to make better choices so you can begin to break your sugar addiction cycle, it is important to have a better understanding of what carbohydrates are and what is meant by terms like, "good carbs, bad carbs, high carbs, low carbs, simple carbs and complex carbs." Well, keep reading and I will help you sort out all those labels in the next chapter.

Chapter 5 - Can You Give Me a Simple Explanation about Carbs?

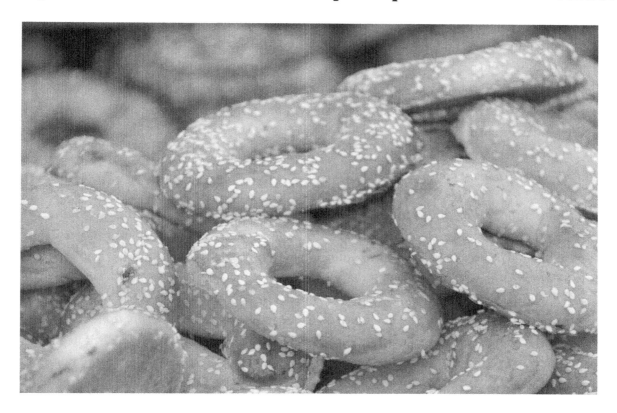

Absolutely! Carbohydrates provide our bodies with energy, and are the major component of the diet in most cultures. They also play an important structural role in the body, making up part of every cell membrane. In addition, the sugar ribose is a crucial part of DNA and RNA, the molecules that enable all living things to pass genetic information to their descendants.

In discussing carbohydrates in our diet, there are three common ways that carbs are divided:

1. Simple carbs and complex carbs

2. Good carbs and bad carbs

3. High carbs and low carbs

Obviously, there is a danger of over-simplifying things, but this is a good starting point for our discussion.

Simple Carbs versus Complex Carbs

The names for these two classifications of carbohydrates make them easy to understand. Moreover, when you finish reading about them, it will not be hard for you to remember which one to focus on when trying to decide what to eat the next time you are hungry.

Simple Carbs

Simple carbs consist of only one or two sugar units strung together. Glucose, the sugar that most commonly circulates in our blood, is a single unit sugar, as is fructose (fruit sugar). Sucrose (table sugar) is a two-unit sugar, made of one glucose and one fructose molecule joined together. Lactose (milk sugar) is another two-unit sugar, made of one galactose unit joined to a glucose unit. All simple sugars supply your body with a quick source of energy, but unlike complex carbs, they are nutritionally empty. This means that they generally have no associated minerals or vitamins, so all they provide is energy. They go into your bloodstream quickly and create spikes in your blood sugar levels. They lack fiber so they seldom satisfy your appetite for any length of time.

Oftentimes, after you eat foods that are simple carbs, you find yourself feeling even hungrier, tired, and actually craving more simple carbs. This is often due to the high spike in your blood sugar levels, followed by a big drop in it. This results in your body feeling exhausted from the hard work it has just gone through in dealing with the sugar hit you gave it.

A few examples of foods made up of simple carbs are: *fruit drinks; corn syrup; table sugar; candy; brown sugar; honey; soft drinks.* Fruit is also in the simple carb category—what makes it healthier for you is not that it is a different kind of sugar, but that the fruit contains fiber, minerals, and vitamins that your body also needs.

Complex Carbs

Complex carbohydrates consist of sugar molecules that are strung together like a long string of beads. To digest them, the body must separate the beads and deal with them one at a time. Since they must be separated into simple sugar units to be absorbed, these sugars are digested much slower than ones categorized as simple carbs. Many of these complex carbs are plant foods that are high in minerals and vitamins. Their ingestion into your system does not cause severe spikes in your blood sugar levels, and they are often high in fiber that helps to satisfy your appetite. It is important to remember, however, that ultimately even complex carbs are broken down into sugars, and the caloric load can be substantial.

Here are a few examples of complex carbohydrates: *green vegetables; starchy vegetables like corn, potatoes, and pumpkin; legumes like peas, lentils, beans, and peanuts.*

While you might think your food choices would mean choosing complex carbs over simple ones every time, it also becomes necessary for you to look at how they are processed. Processing refers to chemical treatments food is subjected to, such as bleaching flour or adding coloring to vegetables to improve appearance, or chemicals added as preservatives. Not all processing is harmless. For instance, white bread is made from a complex carbohydrate, yet it is highly processed; a piece of fruit is a simple carb, yet it is not processed. When it comes to choosing complex carbs versus simple carbs, be sure to look at processed versus unprocessed, too.

Good Carbs versus Bad Carbs

To walk you through this section, we need to come up with a definition to distinguish between good carbs and bad carbs. How about this? We will start by agreeing that good carbs are carbs that are "good" for our bodies.

Good Carbs

When foods are classified as good carbs, here is some of what this label means:

- They consist of foods that work with the mechanics of our bodies

- Good carbs do not put any additional strain on our system when they are being processed within our bodies

- They do not cause side effects like bloating, inflammation, and a host of other negative side effects. This means they are easy to digest and consist mostly of whole foods that are readily found in nature (foods that are minimally processed)

- Our bodies are able to easily extract the vitamins and nutrients found within the makeup of these foods

1. As a rule, good carbs are going to be foods that are minimally processed or not processed at all. They consist of complex carbohydrates—this means they offer our bodies our best fuel sources

2. They offer our bodies good nutrition, resulting in more energy as fuel to keep us going. As one author put it, "It is like making deposits to your body's energy bank account."

3. They tend to be sources of high fiber content that makes them healthy for our bodies. Because of their fiber, these foods are broken down slower in our bodies, resulting in slow, steady rises in blood sugar levels

4. Foods considered good carbs are ones that satisfy our hunger longer and ward off other symptoms like irritability and mood swings

Below is a short list of some good carbs to include in your diet. These are the foods you will want to learn to eat more of in the days, months, and years ahead:

- All kinds of vegetables, especially non-starchy ones

- All kinds of fruits (Be sure to limit the amounts and learn which fruits are lower in sugar, especially if you are trying to lose weight. I'll show you more of how to know this later on.)

- Root vegetables

- Whole-fat dairy products

Bad Carbs

Now for the bad carbs. Bad carbs are pretty much the opposite of good carbs. Below is a short overview of what is meant by the term:

- Bad carbs consist of foods that can be difficult for our bodies to process. This is often because these foods are "man-made" or refined, often resulting in foods our bodies often do not even recognize as food

- Many can cause side effects like bloating, inflammation, headaches, cramping, etc.

- They consist of foods that have little to no nutritional value. If our bodies cannot break down the foods we eat into tiny pieces that they can use, then we will not remain healthy nor will we be able to receive the vital nutrients from foods that are necessary for life.

1. Bad carbs are considered foods that have been processed, had sugars added to them, or our bodies have problems digesting and processing them

2. They offer very little in the way of nutritional value, even to the point that they are often classified as "empty calories." Because of this, bad carbs should be avoided to help keep from adding extra calories into your diet, often resulting in weight gain.

3. A high intake of bad carbs can cause you to not only gain weight, but also cause you to feel hungry, make your blood pressure rise, accelerate your aging process, and even advance cancer growth.

So, what are some sources for bad carbs? Check out this short list:

- Sugar (no surprise about this one)

- All kinds of grains (Grains have a high glycemic index causing spikes in blood sugar levels and other symptoms. Even whole grains cause this)

- Potatoes (They cause spikes of your blood sugar just like processed grains do)

- Sweetened soft drinks

- Processed foods like cookies, cakes, candy, pretzels, and many others

To sum it all up—good carbs are carbs that are good for your body while bad carbs are not!

High Carbs versus Low Carbs

Another way foods are divided is into high carbs versus low carbs.

High Carbs

High carbs, as its name indicates, are foods that have a high sugar content and raise your blood sugar levels quickly and often dramatically. Like the list of foods listed above under simple carbs and bad carbs, these foods should be limited and avoided if possible.

Low Carbs

Low carb foods, however, are ones with a lower sugar content and do not impact your blood levels like high carbs do.

I am sure you have heard about different diets that are low in carbs called "low carb diets." These tend to be healthier than high carb diets because foods that are featured are those with low sugar content. This often means you can eat more of them without experiencing problems with insulin spikes and other issues. Low carb diets are usually combined with high protein and fats to make up a complete eating plan.

Then there are high carb diets. Foods with a high sugar and starch content are the majority of foods consumed on this diet plan. If it seems unlikely that anyone would deliberately choose a diet high in carbs, realize that many low-fat diets are in fact high-carb diets. Since the amount of protein in most diets varies only a little, reducing fat means increasing sugar, unless calories are severely restricted.

There is one other area you need to know about as you start to cut back on sugars in your diet. It has to do with two tools called the Glycemic Index and Glycemic Load and these will be our topic for the next chapter.

Chapter 6 – How Can the Glycemic Index Help with My Sugar Detox?

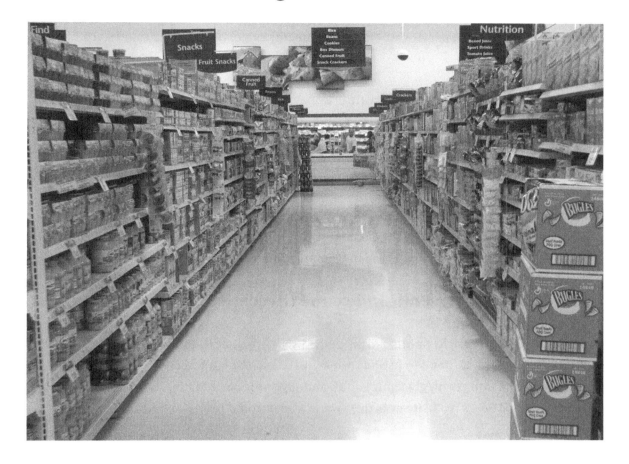

The Glycemic Index (GI) is a system that ranks the effects that foods have on your blood sugar levels when you eat them. In other words, it is a measure of how quickly a carbohydrate gets digested and releases sugar (glucose) into your bloodstream. The Glycemic Index does not take into account the caloric content or the serving size of foods.

The GI compares the effect of a given food to that of ingesting pure glucose, which is rated as 100. If a food has half the effect on blood sugar as glucose has, its GI would be 50. The closer to 100, the quicker and larger the blood sugar change. There are even a few substances that raise the blood sugar more than an equivalent amount of pure glucose, and have a GI greater than 100.

To give you a basic breakdown of how foods are categorized using the GI:

- < 50 is considered low

- 50 – 70 is moderate

- 70+ is considered high because the carbs turn into blood sugar very quickly—create spikes in sugar and insulin

Then there is something called the Glycemic Load (GL). This is a system where foods are rated by the amount of carbohydrates in a serving of that food. For this scale, the number ranges are different from the GI:

- < 10 is considered low and has very little impact on your blood sugar level

- 11 – 19 is moderate and will create spikes in sugar and insulin

- 20+ is considered high and tends to create spikes in your blood sugar levels. Eat sparingly

The consensus among physicians and researchers nowadays is to consult the GL of a food when trying to decide which foods to eat. The goal is to try and pick foods that produce little to moderate spikes in your blood sugar levels—meaning they contain fewer carbs per serving.

Free Download of Glycemic Index and Glycemic Load for Common Foods

(There is a free PDF article published in 2002 by the American Journal of Clinical Nutrition that has a lengthy bunch of foods listing their GI and GL numbers. You can find this at http://tenfingerspublishing.com/glycemic-index-and-glycemic-load-for-foods/. There is also a simpler chart located on Dr. Al Sears' website at http://www.alsearsmd.com/glycemic-index/)

For example, let's say you are trying to cut back on your sugar intake, especially because you are learning that by doing so, it can help you lose weight. You start to feel hungry so you want to eat something healthy. You think, "I would like some fruit. Should I eat some strawberries or a slice of watermelon?"

The GI for strawberries is 40, while the number for watermelon is 72. It sounds like strawberries are the way to go. However, it does not stop there. You also need to see what the GL is for both.

Looking at the numbers from Dr. Sears' website, it shows that strawberries have a GI of 40, but only a GL of 3.6. Watermelon has a GI of 72 and a GL of 7.2. With the serving size based on one-cup for each fruit and using the scale above, it would appear that either one would be a good choice because they both fall below 10 on the GL scale.

As a quick reference for some everyday foods, I have put together a small chart of foods people commonly eat. (These numbers come from the Harvard Health Publication website.)

Glycemic Index of Familiar Foods

Grapefruit	25	Couscous	65
Pear	38	Whole wheat bread	71
Apple	39	Bagel	72
Whole milk	41	Watermelon	72
Bulgur wheat	48	Gatorade®	78
Orange juice	50	White bread	79
Brown rice	54	Puffed wheat cereal	80
Pita bread	57	Rice cakes	82
Grapes	59	White rice	89
Sweet corn on cob	60	Cornflakes	93
Honey	61	French bread	95
Coca Cola®	63	Fruit Roll-Ups®	99
Hamburger bun	61	Baked russet potato	111

Did you happen to notice the last entry—the one for baked russet potato? It is a whopping 111 on the GI scale. That tells you that it raises the blood sugar levels in your bloodstream worse than eating pure glucose does!

Also, notice that grains, which are carbohydrates, have a high GI, especially those grains that contain gluten like wheat, spelt, and kamut—grains I have used in my baking in the past. Because they contain gluten and cause rapid elevations in your bloodstream, I tend to be hesitant to recommend whole grains. Having studied the Paleolithic diet for awhile, I know this is a big reason why grains are not part of that eating style. (But that is a subject for another book.)

As a side note, however, if you consult Dr. Sears' numbers, you will notice that the GL for whole grains is lower than the GL for processed grains as found in white bread. This is because whole grains are not as refined and still contain some of their fiber content.

Additionally, there have been studies conducted that have suggested there may be a link associated between the consistent ingestion of high GI foods and medical conditions such as:

- Heart disease

- High cholesterol

- Type 2 diabetes

- High blood pressure

- Abdominal obesity

Knowing about these two tools and how to read them can empower you to make smart decisions concerning what to eat while you stay focused on your goals. Educating yourself about where foods are ranked on the Glycemic Index and their Glycemic Load will help you choose your foods wisely.

In the next section, I want to help you see some places sugars "hide" in our diet.

Chapter 7 – Where Do Sugars Hide in My Food?

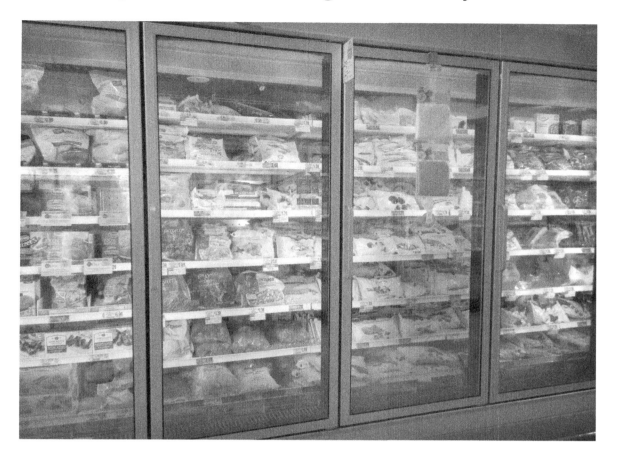

Now that you have learned how to determine the sugar content in foods, I want to help you discover where sugar hides. You will find that sugar hides in places you could easily detect and probably already know about like sodas, candy, and cakes. However, as the last chapter may have helped you see, carbs are also in foods you believed to be healthy, like breads and potatoes.

Much of their "health content" is determined by how they are processed and their serving size, meaning whole grains are "healthier" than processed grains, but they still contain high levels of carbohydrates. Knowing the kinds of foods that naturally contain sugar and ones that have sugar added will also help you learn what to look for when you decide to cut back on your sugar intake.

Places Where Sugar Can Hide

Grain Products	Sweet Treats	Beverages	Condiments and Sauces
Cookies	Candy	Regular soft drinks	Ketchup
Pretzels	Cake	Sports drinks	Barbecue sauce
Cereals	Ice cream	Energy drinks	Salad dressings
Bagels	Pastries	Juice-flavored drinks	Pasta sauces
Bread (whole wheat and white)	Pies	Powdered drink mixes	Gravy
Flours (rice, corn, soy, etc.)	Chocolate	Flavored coffees and teas	Worcestershire sauce
Cakes	Jellies and Jams	Milk shakes	Steak sauces
Donuts	Energy bars	Alcohol	Relish

And believe me when I tell you that this list could go on and on! I am sure no one is surprised that jellies and jams have lots of sugars, but barbecue sauce and salad dressing? Sometimes, it seems like sugar is added for no good reason—and there are times when it is added for texture more than for taste. And the calories keep adding up!

What Other Names Are There for Sugar?

While we are on the subject of sugar hiding in foods, it is also necessary to learn the various names for sugar. Many can be found in products you already consume or are tempted to try. Discovering their names and where they hide means becoming acquainted with the different names for sugar.

For example, barley malt is a type of sugar; however, if you did not know this, you would not realize that ingesting a product that uses barley malt as a sweetener is going to cause your blood sugar levels to spike.

This is a long list of names--some you will already know, while others will surprise you, and the list includes ones you have never heard of. Some of these occur naturally in foods like fruits and milk while others are added during processing.

I have tried to group them by similar sounding names so you can start to see the patterns like "syrup" and words ending in "o-s-e."

The Many Names for Sugar

Sugar	Demerara sugar	Lactose	Agave nectar
Brown sugar	Muscovado sugar	Glucose	Fruit nectars (pear, peach, apricot, etc.)
Date sugar	Sucanat	Maltose	Barley malt
Cane sugar	High fructose corn syrup	Sucrose	Rapadura
Palm sugar	Maple syrup	Galactose	Xylitol
Raw cane sugar	Brown rice syrup	Fruit juice	Sorbitol
Confectioner's powdered sugar	Corn syrup	Cane juice	Mannitol
Invert sugar	Malt syrup	Evaporated cane juice	Stevia
Beet sugar	Sorghum syrup	Maltodextrin	Evaporated corn sweetener
Coconut sugar	Fructose	Honey	Fruit juice concentrate
Turbinado sugar	Dextrose	Molasses	I'm sure I forgot one ☺

I suppose I may have missed a few, but I think this will give you a good start for investigating sugars in your foods the next time you go shopping. This leads me to point out a few things about the Nutrition Facts Label you will end up reading on a product's packaging.

Nutrition Facts Labeling of Sugar

When you look at the labeling on food products, you need to look at the "total carbohydrate" number—not just the sugar listing. This number is made from a combination of the other entries—dietary fiber, sugars and sometimes sugar alcohols. Because carbs are also contained in grain products, natural or added sugars are only part of the equation.

Food labeling can be tricky to say the least. Let me give you a few examples:

- When a product says, "less sugar" or "reduced sugar," it actually means the sugar has been "reduced" by at least 25% in this product compared to a product of similar ingredients. (Just because a product is labeled, "reduced sugar" does not mean it is lower in calories. Sometimes extra fat and carbohydrates are added to offset or balance out the taste due to lack of sugar)

- When you see, "no added sugar," it does NOT mean that there is not any sugar in the product; it means no sugar-containing ingredients were added during processing. However, a product may still be high in carbohydrates due to its content

- If a package reads, "sugar free," that actually means there is less than .05 grams per serving as indicated on the label. It means there are not any natural sugars present and no sugar was added; however, you still have to check the label for the total number of carbohydrates— "sugar-free does not mean it is carb-free."

- When a package has an entry for "sugar alcohols" (Xylitol, mannitol, and sorbitol are all common sugar alcohols added as sweeteners), realize that many of these foods still contain calories and carbohydrates. Along with fiber, sugar alcohols do not affect your blood sugar levels like other carbohydrates because as a "food," they are not completely absorbed into your system. However, be aware that their side effects often consist of intestinal gas, bloating and diarrhea.

Added sugars for a product are listed down in the "ingredient list" at the bottom of the Nutrition Facts Label. As of this writing, there is not an "added sugars" line inserted under the "Sugars" section of the label so you have to read the ingredients to actually find out what you are consuming.

A product can have a lot of sugar in it because a manufacturer often breaks up the total amount of sugar among several different ingredients. If a product contains 20 grams of sugar, many are choosing to use 10 grams of one kind of sugar, 5 grams of another, and still 5 grams of a third kind of sugar. Because ingredients are listed from "most ingredients used" down to "least amounts used," your product can have a lot of sugar in it without you noticing—unless you have learned the various names for sugar.

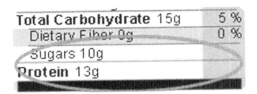

Total Carbohydrate 15g	5 %
Dietary Fiber 0g	0 %
Sugars 10g	
Protein 13g	

Total Carbohydrate 46g	15 %
Dietary Fiber Less than 1g	3 %
Sugars 44g	
Protein 9g	

Notice the two images above. They are for the same kind of product. The one on the left contains sugars that naturally occur in the product. The image on the right has "added sugars." The only way you are going to know the difference is to read the ingredients' list below this labeling. It certainly would be helpful if there were a line inserted in the "total carbohydrate" section that said "added sugars." Maybe someday…

While we are looking at labels, do not forget another common trick, the "serving size" ploy. The small bottle of fruit drink looks like it "only" has 30 grams of sugar in it. But wait! The manufacturer says that the twelve-ounce bottle contains two servings—and *each* serving has 30 grams of sugar. Unless you shared your bottle of juice, you just drank down 60 grams of sugar!

Chapter 8- What Exactly Is a Sugar Detox?

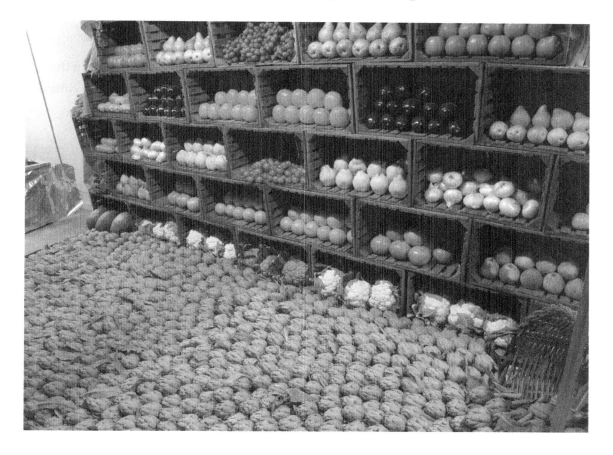

As you have learned by now, sugars can have a detrimental effect on your body. We have discussed what sugar is, where it hides, and the damage it can do. Now that you have read this far, you may be thinking about doing a sugar detox because you have discovered some of the harmful things sugar can do—and may have done--to your body. With this goal in mind, let me help you understand what this means.

According to the Cambridge Dictionary, a detox consists of "a period of time when you stop ingesting harmful and unhealthy drugs, drinks, and foods so that your health will improve." That is a definition that is not difficult to understand, so let's move on.

What steps are involved in conducting a sugar detox? Well, on paper, they are really quite simple:

- First, you remove foods high in sugars and carbs from your home, and minimize them in your diet as well.

- Secondly, you learn about and concentrate on eating only those foods that are low in their sugar content and you promise yourself you will not add any extra sugar to your food.

- Thirdly, if you "fall of the wagon," you start the period of your detox over again—some say starting over with Day 1. I would say pick up where you left off. Do not beat yourself up, refocus and get going again.

There are some detox programs that last for 3 days, 21 days, and even 30 days. While these have an end in sight, I would say that the "ultimate" period of time for eliminating or drastically cutting back on sugar would be for as long as you can—maybe even for life.

One of the big reasons for doing a detox is to educate yourself concerning how sugar affects you. You can discover this by noticing how you feel, what symptoms you experience or which ones disappear, and what you notice differently about yourself when the actual "test" period is over. As you add sugars back into your diet, symptoms may reappear. If you never make the effort and take the time to eliminate sugars from your diet, you will not notice anything different from what you are experiencing now. Changes in your mood, the way your body feels, your mental clarity, and many other improvements can result if you try detoxing for a little while. Personally, if I had not detoxed from sugar for 30 days, I would not have realized that when I do have some sugar on occasion, this is what makes my index finger joints achy and swollen. It is like my personal built-in barometer of knowing when I have had too much sugar recently.

Now, do not misunderstand me. While "on paper" it looks simple—in practice it can be quite difficult. As we have talked about already, sugar is everywhere! It is not an easy thing to get away from. It takes awareness and commitment to even accomplish eliminating sugar for one day!

However, if you decide to give a sugar detox a try, something wonderful can happen just by taking the time to educate yourself about sugar—contemplating a sugar detox will increase your awareness of what sugar is, what names it is called by, where it hides, and how to find healthier alternatives to eating it.

According to a report published by the Department of Health and Human Resources:

"Two hundred years ago, the average American ate only 2 pounds of sugar a year. In 1970, we ate 123 pounds of sugar per year. Today, the average American consumes almost 152 pounds of sugar in one year. This is equal to 3 pounds (or 6 cups) of sugar consumed in one week!"

And listen to this statistic from the same study:

"Nutritionists suggest that Americans should get only 10% of their calories from sugar. This equals 13.3 teaspoons of sugar per day (based on 2,000 calories per day). The current average is 42.5 teaspoons of sugar per day!"

So how much do you think you consume each day? You probably do not know for sure, and if you had to guess, you would probably underestimate how much sugar you really consume. Why not, just for fun, consider writing down what you ate today or yesterday, as best you can remember, and see if you can calculate how much sugar you consumed. I think you will be surprised at how much of that "white stuff" you actually put into your body.

Chapter 9 – How Do I Begin a Sugar Detox?

First, you have to want to do a sugar detox program for YOU! Your decision has to be motivated by your desire to want to take better care of yourself—to make a healthier you—to be better physically than you are right now. It has to be a decision that YOU own—something you know is best for you. If you think you want to do this because your friend did it and had great success with it, that can be a good reason to consider it; however, you have to own your decision.

Your decision to do a sugar detox has to be something within yourself that gets you excited about the possibilities of life with less sugar in it because you may experience some rough spots and struggles. Therefore, know why you are doing this by writing down your goals and know what is motivating you. Then, put these somewhere where you can see them everyday.

Beginning a sugar detox is one of the easiest—and hardest decisions to make. It is easy because you can decide to do it at any time. It is difficult because sugar is more addictive than you think. As you may remember from the quiz I had you take when you first started this book, sugar can even seem to have some mystical powers over us. It tests our willpower, it seems to "call our name," and it can even cause us to be sneaky and secretive about consuming it. Here are two huge reasons why this is so:

- Some researchers claim sugar can be just as addictive as cocaine

- Whenever you eat sugar, it causes the release of dopamine in your brain—a chemical known for controlling your sense of pleasure that in turn affects your moods

My purpose in sharing these things is so you will realize why eliminating sugar can be difficult. This type of detoxing is almost like going through drug rehabilitation—sugar can be that addicting! Once again, knowing what you are getting into will help you be prepared.

A Short Disclaimer

For the remainder of this book, I want to provide you with a lifelong plan for eliminating sugars from your diet. These are guidelines and plans for you to use once you have made up your mind to do it. I will present you with how you can begin, things you will experience as you start, what you can expect to feel while you are detoxing, and some action points for maintaining a lifestyle of cutting back on sugar in your life.

Occasionally, you WILL eat added sugars off and on for the rest of your life. Just know this and do not beat yourself up over it when you do. However, I do hope that after you have experienced a detox of sugar that you will be able to stop voluntarily, sooner than you might have in the past, and that you even find it easier to do each time it happens.

Be sure to consult your physician if you are diabetic or have problems with blood sugar issues like insulin resistance. Also, consult your physician if you are on medications that help control your blood sugar.

Time to Begin

1. One of the first things you will want to decide is WHEN will you begin your detox and HOW LONG it will last.

- Take a moment to check your calendar to see if you have a crazy schedule staring you in the face. I do not know about you, but when I have a crazy week, one of the first things to disappear from my life is cooking healthy meals and eating right like I know I should.

- How many days do you want to attempt? If this is your first try, you may want to start with a short period of time, then try longer ones in the future.

- Will you be traveling out of town soon? Being away from home can limit the type of food choices you have.

These are just a few questions to get you thinking so you can plan for success.

2. Be kind to yourself! Take things slowly. Remember, even though you may be preparing for a detox that is limited in time, you also want to make the kind of changes you can see yourself sticking with for a long time. If you have had crummy eating habits for a long time, you may find some aspects of eliminating sugar to be difficult. This is a huge reason why you want to log everything you eat and what you are experiencing when you eat it in your food journal. (Something I will help you set up in a couple of chapters.) While you may slip, you will be able to see victories along the way that can help keep you motivated as well as helping you see areas that cause you to stumble.

Keep in mind throughout your detox that if you mess up, it does not mean you are a failure, that you are worthless or lazy. Who you are is NOT affected by how much sugar you eat or don't eat. If you stumble, try again. Remember, your health is worth fighting for and sugar detoxing can be exactly that—a FIGHT! Not always easy, but definitely worth it!

3. Take an inventory of your refrigerator and pantry. In order to achieve success, you want to make your living environment as "sugar free" as possible. You see, if it is not in your house or apartment, then you have to make a conscious decision to go out and purchase it before you eat it. This alone often gives you time to change your mind and refocus on your goals.

Making your environment sugar free means you will need to eliminate sugars that are obvious—cookies, candy, cake, ice cream and other products like these. You will also need to eliminate food items like pasta, sodas, white bread and fruit juice (I do love the taste of orange juice.)

4. Make sure you have a good understanding of how to read food labels for when you go shopping. Knowing some of the more common names for sugar will help you tremendously because you will be able to spot them, despite their names. In addition, although fruits in the produce section do not have product labels on them, remember this basic rule for helping you decide what to buy: the sweeter a fruit tastes is a good indicator that it will have a high sugar content. FYI--Bananas actually increase in their sugar content the riper they get.

5. Decide right now to give yourself some kind of reward when you have finished your sugar detox, but try not to make it food. Reward yourself with something like a new outfit; an appointment to pamper yourself at a spa or nail salon; take a day trip to someplace you have been wanting to go; buy a new book; meet with friends to go shopping. There are many wonderful treats you can give yourself once you have finished your detox. You may even find that these can motivate you to get through rough spots you may encounter.

Foods for Your Detox

Here I have listed the main categories of foods with some of the specific kinds named that you are allowed to eat on most sugar detox programs. Later you will find a grocery list that contains these foods so you can print it out and take it with you when you go shopping. This part may seem overwhelming, but it is part of the process to help you learn how to eat better with less sugar.

Meats: Most every kind is allowed because meats are proteins and do not contain carbohydrates. The problem with meat is when sugars are added through sauces and condiments. Also, do not buy processed meats because they often have sugar added at the manufacturer.

Vegetables: You want to pick vegetables that are low in carbohydrates. Liberally enjoy vegetables like lettuces, peppers, onions, tomatoes, asparagus, cauliflower, broccoli, cucumbers, celery, zucchini, and others like them. You can do some research on vegetables that are low on the GI and the GL scale and are not starchy.

Remember that **starch = sugar.** Avoid vegetables like potatoes, most squashes, corn, and peas because they do have a high-starch content. NOTE: Be sure to check the packaging on frozen vegetables—they often contain added sugar!

Fruit: The best fruits to eat when you are detoxing are the ones that have almost no natural sugars. That means, they are going to be the ones that are on the sour end of the fruit family—lemons, limes, and grapefruits. Try to stay at "25" or below on the Glycemic Index for this category.

Dairy: You want your dairy products to contain the natural fats found in milk because the fat slows down the effects of lactose (sugar) in your bloodstream when you eat them. Quantity needs to be limited, as every eight ounces of milk contains 12 grams of sugar. Concentrate on foods like whole milk, plain yogurt and kefir, heavy cream, cottage cheese, and aged cheeses. (The aging process helps bring the lactose levels in the milk almost down to zero.)

Nuts and Seeds: Nuts, seeds, and the butters created with them are healthy fats. They contain little if any carbohydrates. Just make sure that if you buy them already processed that there is no added sugar in them. Experiment and enjoy foods like pumpkin and sunflower seeds, almonds and almond butter, unsweetened coconut, macadamias, walnuts, pecans, hazelnuts, and seeds like hemp, chia, and flax.

Fats and Oils: Fats do not contain any carbohydrates at all so they are good to use in cooking, in salads, and for seasonings. Some of the healthiest are grass-fed butter, avocado oil, sesame oil, extra virgin olive oil, and animal fats like beef and duck. I would also encourage you to cook with coconut oil if you currently do not. It will not burn like many oils do at higher temperatures (like olive oil) and it is very good for you.

Beverages: This area will seem very limiting when you are detoxing. That is because there are very few beverages we are used to drinking that do not contain added sugars. Ones that you will be free to enjoy are water, black coffee, unsweetened teas, club soda, mineral and seltzer water, and unsweetened nut milks.

So, now you see what the foods look like with a sugar detox. At first, this may seem extremely limiting, and it certainly is especially if you currently eat many sugary foods. At least you now have a better idea of what is involved.

In the next chapter, I have put together a fairly comprehensive list of foods you can buy at the store so you are prepared for your detox. It is a compilation of several different detox programs so some items may or may not be included in the detox program you decide to do.

Chapter 10 – What Does a Grocery List Look Like?

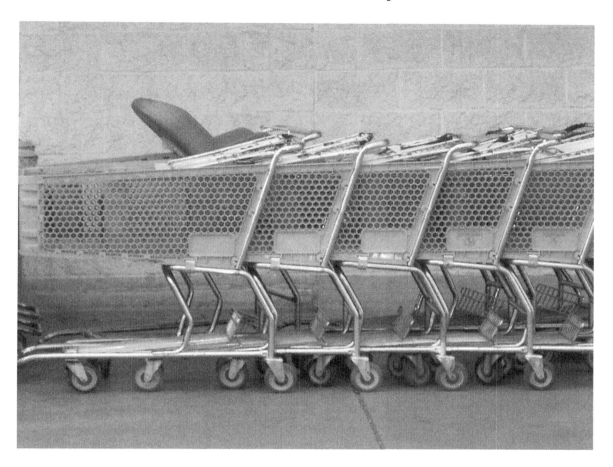

Like many of you, I want life to be as simple as it can be so when I was busy trying to think of what would help you prepare for a detox program, I wanted to provide you with some helpful tools. The best one I could come up with for this section was a grocery list filled with the items that are "legal" for most detox programs whose focus is to eliminate and cut back on sugar.

I have inserted a list of these foods below. For your convenience, you are free to go to http://tenfingerspublishing.com/detox-grocery-list-for-sugar-detoxification/ and download the PDF of this list so you can have your own personal copy to take with you to the store.

A Word of Caution: Remember, in the beginning, you definitely want to limit fruits--even the ones that are LOW in carbs and have numbers on the Glycemic Index below 25 and less than 10 as their Glycemic Load. However, I have included them in the chart below because I also wanted this to be a grocery list you could use after your detox so you will have a list of healthier foods.

Meat	Seafood	Vegetables	
Beef	Catfish	Artichoke	Lettuce
Bison	Carp	Asparagus	Mushrooms
Boar	Clams	Arugula	Mustard greens
Buffalo	Grouper	Beets	Okra
Chicken	Halibut	Bok Choy	Onions
Duck	Herring	Broccoli	Parsley
Eggs	Lobster	Brussels Sprouts	Parsnip
Game	Mackerel	Cabbage	Peppers
Goat	Mahi Mahi	Carrots	Radicchio
Goose	Mussels	Cassava	Radish
Lamb	Oysters	Cauliflower	Rapini
Mutton	Salmon	Celery	Rutabaga
Pork	Sardines	Chard	Seaweed
Quail	Scallops	Collards	Shallots
Rabbit	Shrimp	Cucumber	Snap peas
Squab	Snail	Daikon	Spinach
Turkey	Snapper	Dandelion	Squash
Veal	Swordfish	Eggplant	Sugar snaps
Venison	Trout	Endive	Sweet potato

Nuts and Seeds		Vegetables (cont.)	
		Fennel	Taro
Almonds	Pistachios	Garlic	Tomatillios
Brazil nuts	Poppy seeds	Green beans	Tomato
Chestnuts	Pumpkin seeds	Green onions	Turnip greens
Hazelnuts	Sesame seeds	Jicama	Turnips
Macadamias	Sunflower seeds	Kale	Watercress
Pecans	Walnuts	Kohlrabi	Yam
Pine nuts		Leeks	Yucca

Fats and Oils		Fruits	
Avocado	Ghee (clarified butter)	Apples (green/tart)	Melon*
Avocado oil	Lard	Apricot*	Nectarines*
Bacon fat	Macadamia nut oil	Banana*	Oranges*
Butter	Olive oil	Blackberries*	Papaya*
Chicken fat	Palm oil/shortening	Blueberries*	Passion fruit*
Coconut oil	Tallow	Cantaloupe*	Peaches*
Coconut milk	Sesame oil	Cherries* (sour for detox)	Pears*
Duck fat	Walnut oil	Cranberries (raw)	Persimmon*

Beverages			
Almond milk	Herbal tea (unsweetened)	Dates*	Pineapple*
Coconut milk	Mineral water	Figs*	Plantain*
Coconut water	Water	Grapefruit	Plums*
Coffee (black)		Grapes*	Pomegranate*

Guava*	Raspberries*
Kiwi*	Rhubarb
Lemon	Star fruit
Lime	Strawberries*
Lychee*	Tangerine*
Mango*	Watermelon*

A Note about Fruits:

In the fruit section, the ones with an asterisk (*) after them are foods you should wait to eat after your detox.

As a general rule, the sweeter the fruit, the higher the sugar content. Plus, the riper a fruit becomes, the higher the sugar content. Example: Better to eat a banana that is firm and not very ripe to keep the sugar content down.

Herbs & Spices			
Anise	Cilantro	Juniper berry	Peppermint
Annato	Cinnamon	Lavender	Rosemary
Basil	Clove	Lemongrass	Saffron
Bay leaf	Coriander	Lemon verbena	Spearmint
Caraway	Cumin	Licorice	Star anise
Cardamom	Curry	Mace	Tarragon
Carob	Dill	Marjoram	Thyme
Cayenne	Fennel	Mint	Turmeric
Celery seed	Fenugreek	Mustard	Vanilla
Chervil	Galangal	Oregano	Wasabi
Chicory	Garlic	Paprika	Za'atar
Chili peppers	Ginger	Parsley	
Chives	Horseradish	Pepper, black	

As you can see, this list is more extensive than you may have originally thought it would be. And if you are like me, there are foods on this list that I still have never tried so there is still some room for experimentation.

Free Download of Grocery List

Once again, if you would like to have a PDF print out of this for your shopping trips and easy reference at home, just go to http://tenfingerspublishing.com/detox-grocery-list-for-sugar-detoxification/ and download a copy whenever you need one. I hope this encourages you and helps you get off to a great start.

Chapter 11- Now That I Know What to Buy, What's Next?

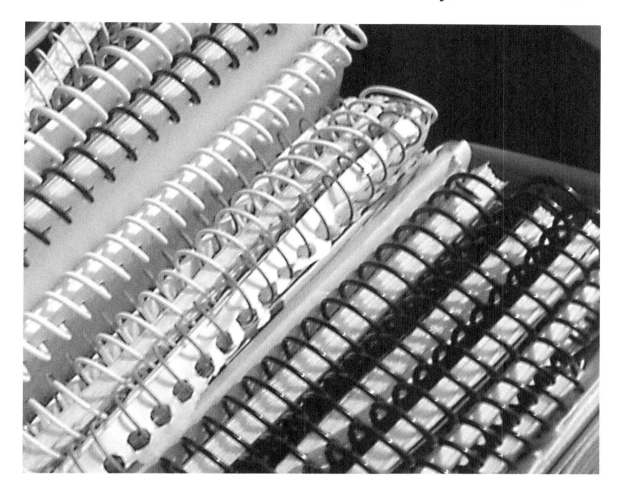

Now that you have read this far, you are probably asking, "Now what?" I would suggest you start by analyzing the things you currently eat on a regular basis, how you believe they affect your body, what changes you are willing to make, and how long do you want to attempt a detox. Ultimately, the final question should be, "Can I see myself cutting back on sugar for the rest of my life?"

While this may be too far out in the distant future for you to think about now, that is fine. However, the last question is an important one to keep in the back of your mind because you are ultimately working toward making "life changes." You will proceed in that direction by taking small, yet deliberate steps and changes along the way as you discover how your body, moods, and attitudes are changed and affected when sugar is greatly decreased.

If you have decided you are ready to make some changes, find a notebook and let's get started…

Now, with your notebook, pen or pencil, or your computer like I do with this assignment, let's begin with setting up your food journal.

How to Set Up a Food Journal

Keeping a food journal keeps you honest. It has been proven that most people underestimate what they eat in a day if they do not write it down. Since you are working toward making changes in your eating habits, a food journal can help you tremendously.

1. Begin by writing down everything you can think of that you eat on a regular basis that has sugar in it.

2. Put a question mark by the ones you are not sure about but suspect may have added sugar. You can check later to see if you are right or not

3. You want to create spaces that will allow you to record the following:

   - Date

   - Time

   - Foods Eaten

   - Place - Where you were when you ate: at home, in a restaurant, a friend's house, etc.

   - How much

   - Beverage

   - Feelings – What you were feeling when you decided to eat: real hunger, loneliness, sadness, etc.

   - Activity level – Had you been exercising, sitting for long periods, driving, awoke from sleeping, etc.

   - End of the day

Feel free to put anything else you think you will want to track in your journal. You can even keep track of your weight weekly.

4. Make yourself record what you eat in your journal when you eat it. Also, be specific. State food items individually like, "2 pieces of whole wheat bread, tomato, lettuce, and 2 ounces of roast beef," along with condiments like pickles and mustard, rather than simply writing, "a roast beef sandwich." Oh, and do not forget to record your snacks, too.

5. Be sure to log the time, date, and where you ate. Taking the time to keep track of these things may help you see patterns in how close your meals are to each other, indicating whether you are under eating or overeating, and if you tend to eat more when you are watching television or eating out with friends in a restaurant. This can be a valuable tool for discovering any routines in your eating habits you may not have even been aware of.

6. Be honest about your feelings when you decide to eat. Because many people eat for reasons other than hunger, tracking your feelings can help you see why you eat and what you choose to eat.

7. Quantities of food are important to write down. When you have to quantify your food amounts, it makes you more aware of how much, or how little you are actually eating.

8. Record your beverages, too. It is important to track what you drink throughout the day. Many people do not realize how many calories they consume in their liquids. Additionally, writing down what you drink when you eat may help you see patterns here as well. For instance, somewhere along the way, I started drinking orange juice when I eat popcorn, which is not very often. However, whenever I do eat popcorn, I feel like I have to have orange juice with my popcorn. It is now such an automatic pairing of foods for me that I seldom eat popcorn when we go out to the movies. (I am still looking for a movie theater near me that sells orange juice.)

9. Write down your physical activity. Be sure to record what, if any, physical activity you did during the day and for how long. This will often affect what you eat and how much as well.

10. Record your thoughts and impressions at the end of each day. Do your best to only record positive thoughts here. Look for your victories. Record even the smallest ones—just make sure they are positive comments.

11. Promise yourself you will keep a food journal for at least 30 days. Keeping a journal for at least a month gives you time, and your body time, to notice changes in what you are eating, how much, when, and how you feel. It will indicate how you eat during the week as opposed to the weekends. It will help you find patterns that otherwise may have gone unnoticed.

At this point, you have probably decided how long you want to try a sugar detox. With your food journal in hand, your pantry and refrigerator sugar free and your grocery shopping list, the next thing you need to do is to develop a plan for eating.

Eat breakfast!

1. I know you have probably heard this many times, because it happens to be true. After you have been asleep all night, your body basically shuts down by going into starvation mode—when your metabolism slows down so it doesn't use up too much of your reserves. Even though you know mentally that you will eat sometime after you wake up, your body does not know that. It shifts into starvation mode because it has no idea if it will be getting any more nourishment. This is a big reason why it is important for you to feed it soon after waking so it can kick back up into high gear.

2. It is best to try to eat something within 30 minutes to 1 hour upon rising—preferably proteins and fats. This is important because your blood levels have fallen dramatically during the night and you need to eat something fairly soon so you do not have problems with low sugar levels. If you put off eating, you can get shaky, irritable, and end up grabbing something sugary instead.

3. Breakfast should consist of foods like eggs (these are not dairy—they are protein), some healthy fats like cheese and nut butters, and possibly some fresh fruit. Be very careful about fruit juices. They are high in carbohydrates so it is generally better to eat the fruit itself. A small 8-ounce glass of orange juice contains 26 grams of sugar!

4. When enjoying bacon for breakfast, try to find a brand that doesn't include nitrites and nitrates in their processing. These additives are still questionable nutritionally so try to avoid them. By doing so, you will have a meat with some fat in it that will sustain your energy levels and suppress your appetite effectively until lunchtime.

5. Additionally, rethink your ideas about breakfast. There are many wonderful foods, as you saw from the food list I gave you for your detox that you could learn to eat for breakfast. Instead of sugary cereals and bagels, try leftovers from dinner, a hamburger patty, and even a bacon, lettuce, and tomato sandwich—using the lettuce in place of bread. While I am not advocating that you give up bread completely, just remember that it is high in carbs, and your goal is to be very mindful of your carb intake.

6. Here are some other breakfast ideas you may want to try:

   - A green smoothie for breakfast using coconut water, lettuce, avocado and tomato

   - An omelet with green pepper, onion, mushrooms, and aged shredded cheddar

   - Scrambled eggs with bacon

- Deviled eggs using avocado as part of the filling

- Greek yogurt with chopped pecans

- With breakfasts, once you think outside the box, your options are endless!

Plan for Healthy Snacks

To get through your detox successfully, you need to have some healthy snacks planned. Consider some of these as options:

- Beef jerky without sugar

- Aged cheddar slices with dill pickle slices

- An occasional green apple (tartness means less sugar) with nut butter

- Homemade trail mix (consider making it without peanuts—these are legumes)

- Greek yogurt with nuts and fresh berries

- A hamburger patty topped with fresh salsa

- Celery stalks spread with almond butter

Take Time to Plan Your Main Meals

Dinners and even lunches are important to plan. You do not want to get to 5 o'clock in the afternoon and realize you have not planned or cooked anything for dinner. These moments will get you into trouble, because it will be difficult to remain with your detox program if you do not have your meal planned. Last-minute meals tend to be high in sugars and carbs—pasta, rice, "helpers" and other quick to fix staples will wreck your detox.

1. The best approach to planning these meals is to think about each meal containing a healthy protein (meat and dairy) that makes up about one-third of your plate, and a low-carb vegetable dish seasoned with butter, herbs and spices to make up the other two-thirds of your meal (steamed veggies or a salad). Once you bring back other fruits into your diet after your detox, these will be options for you to choose from as well.

2. Try to plan meals several days at a time. This will help you be organized when you shop so you have everything you need to be successful.

3. Be sure to make extra servings when you prepare your meals so you can have them as leftovers for lunches and even breakfast.

4. Here are a few ideas for some delicious lunches and dinners:

   - Spaghetti squash topped with sautéed peppers, onions, mushrooms, tomatoes and a protein like chicken, shrimp or beef strips

   - A crockpot full of vegetable beef stew

   - Tuna over a bed of lettuce, tomatoes, bell peppers, onions, mushrooms, nuts, and aged shredded cheese, topped with olive oil and balsamic vinegar

   - Beef and broccoli stir-fry, made with coconut aminos instead of soy sauce

   - Lettuce topped with a few green apple bits, pecans, fresh strawberry slices, and fresh blueberries

These are just a few ideas to get you started. Near the end of this book, I will offer you a link that goes to some recipes you can try as you are detoxing and for times after you are finished.

Chapter 12 – What Are Some Positive and Negative Effects of a Detox?

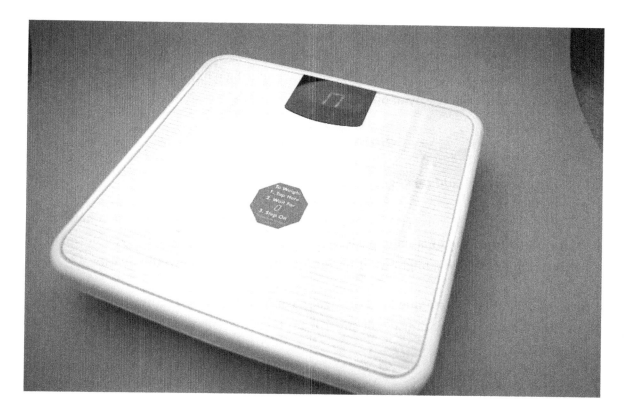

I will be honest and tell you that when you first start your detox, you may not feel very good. Some of what you may experience will have to do with how much detoxing your body will be going through. Most all of these symptoms are mostly bothersome rather than anything dangerous to your health.

Here is a short list of some of the main symptoms you might experience as you begin:

- Tiredness, even flu-like symptoms

- Trouble sleeping

- Feeling like you need extra caffeine to achieve energy

- Headaches

- Dizziness and light-headedness

- Irritability

- Mild dehydration

- Body aches

- Cravings for sugar

For almost everyone who starts a detox, days one through three are the worst. This is because your body is going, "Hey! What's up? Where is the sugar I am used to getting for fuel? What am I supposed to use now?" While I tease, of course, your body is clearly wondering what happened. You will have to give it time to adjust and learn a new way of operating.

Some Detox FAQ's

Should I do a sugar detox "cold turkey?"

This is difficult to answer correctly for everyone because so much depends upon how much sugar you are accustomed to eating on a daily basis. If after taking inventory of what you normally eat, and discover that it is quite a lot, you might want to consider detoxing at a slow, steady rate.

For instance, try to eliminate one kind of sugar each day for a week rather than all at once. It has been shown that people who withdraw all sugar from their diet all at once (grains, fruits, and dairy) often cannot sustain it.

A good strategy would be to take a week or so before you schedule a detox by purposing to slowly eliminate sugar. Change your breakfast from cereal to eggs and other proteins, have a healthy salad for lunch with proteins in it like chicken, tuna, or beef and purpose to eat a nutritious dinner. Most of all, try not to eat anything too sugary for a dessert.

Once you feel as if you have made some good progress, pick a sugar detox program that is not any longer than three days. The odds are you will be successful and this will build your confidence to try another one in the future and one that is longer in duration.

Will I feel crummy during a detox?

Whenever you dramatically change your way of eating, bodily changes are going to occur. In this situation, if you have been used to eating a lot of sugar, your body has been using sugar instead of fat to fuel your body. Consequently, when you take away the sugar, your body has to go through its own transitional process and turn to stored fat for fuel instead. For some this is a rather "painless" transition while for others, their transition may cause them to experience numerous symptoms.

Additionally, I shared with you earlier how some researchers have likened sugar as being as addictive as cocaine so whenever humans withdraw from a drug as powerful as this, there are bound to be some noticeable symptoms.

Something you may not have known before is a high-carb diet can actually cause your body to retain water. There are numerous medical reasons for this but a simple explanation would be simply that when you eat a lot of sugar, your kidneys react by storing salt in your bloodstream instead of letting it pass through. In response, your body has to hang on to any extra fluid it can find to offset the rise in salt content. Consequently, when you cut back on your carbs, your body responds by releasing the salt and water it was holding on to.

How long do the negative types of symptoms last?

Like most issues concerning our bodies, everyone's body tends to respond slightly differently to the same process. For some, these symptoms may start by the end of the first day and can last for three to four days. However, for others, these same symptoms can last for as long as two weeks. There is just no way to tell ahead of time until you have already started with your detox program.

If I end up feeling awful, is there anything I can do to alleviate the symptoms?

Remember you are dealing with fluctuating blood sugar levels in your bloodstream so it makes sense to try to keep these levels as healthy, and as steady as possible. Here are a few tips that may help you get through this transition of high carbs to low carbs as gently as possible:

- Do not go long periods of time without eating. I do not know about you, but whenever I am doing a detox, food is what I think about a lot! I find myself looking forward to when I get to, or should eat again. It is hard to say what is exactly right for you—this is one big reason why you are keeping a food journal. A good rule of thumb, especially in the beginning, is to try to eat something every three hours. By doing so, this should help your blood sugar levels to remain fairly constant, thus avoiding noticeable spikes and dips that cause shakiness and irritability.

- Be sure to drink water often. Because you may experience some of the mild dehydration I mentioned above, you will want to replace these fluids with adequate water, water with lemon, or unsweetened herbal teas. By doing so, you will help yourself ward off headaches that often result when dehydration sets in.

- If possible, make time for rest periods during the day. If tiredness and fatigue are two of the symptoms that happen to you, you will not want to be experiencing a hectic schedule during your detox. If you can, make time during your day to put your feet up and relax for a few minutes. Take a power nap if time allows. Also, back off from a lot of physical activity like strenuous exercising. Instead, turn to walking and other light exercises during this time of detox.

- Be sure to eat healthy fats with your meals. Your body needs extra fuel now that you have taken away the sugar and a great way to do this is to supply it with fat. Our bodies were designed to be fat-burning machines and that is how they run most efficiently. Start using coconut oil in your cooking; drizzle olive oil over your salads and vegetables; melt a tablespoon of butter on your steamed vegetables to add flavor. Especially now, try to add an additional 1 to 2 tablespoons of healthy fats at each meal.

- As with any change in lifestyle, talk to your healthcare professional, especially if you are on any medications. Some of your symptoms may be related to medications you are on and both you and your doctor will want to know how your sugar detoxing and the combination of your medications is affecting you.

What about artificial sweeteners?

Artificial sweeteners are NOT the answer. Not only are they "unnatural," but they also have been found to trick your body into believing it is consuming something sweet. The problem with replacing sugar with artificial sweeteners is this is not teaching you anything new. The goal for your detox and for your life going forward is to retrain your taste buds and your brain by consuming foods that are good for you.

Additionally, studies continue to show troubling side effects with many of the artificial sweeteners on the market. Therefore, if you find yourself needing something sweet, go for a piece of fruit or vegetables like carrots and sweet potatoes even when you are detoxing. While these foods may not be "allowed" during your detoxing period, it is better to consume something healthy and get back on board rather than put chemicals into your body that could harm you.

Will I lose weight?

As I shared with you before, part of what happens during a detox is a mild form of dehydration because your body is releasing fluids that have been held captive. Therefore, you may find that you lose some of those fluids that cause the scale to go down. Logically, if you are making the switch over to eating healthier and filling up on good calories that satisfy and make your body work more efficiently, you may very well lose a few pounds. However, realize that losing weight should not be your primary motivation for a detox, but rather a welcome "by product."

Positive Effects of a Sugar Detox

While there may certainly be some symptoms you experience that are not pleasant, several symptoms that may result can greatly benefit your health and your attitude. Let me share a few with you right now to encourage you in your detox efforts.

Making a decision to detox can have a very empowering effect on you. Anytime you take control of your life, as is required when you rid your body of sugar, demonstrates that you are in control. It shows you that you are willing to face the effects and the addictiveness of sugar head on and make some positive changes. By choosing to overcome the addictive effects of sugar on your body, you offer yourself some of the positive benefits that have been shown to happen when sugar is eliminated from our diets:

1. Better blood sugar and insulin levels ~ As soon as you begin to take sugars out of your diet, your body will respond in positive ways. No longer will you experience dramatic spikes and dips in your blood sugar levels that used to cause you to shake, feel light-headed, and irritable because now your levels will remain more constant. In addition, because your bloodstream will not have an overabundance of sugar in it, your pancreas will not have to respond with such urgency and spill out insulin to bring things under control as it used to.

2. Experience increased levels of energy ~ As your blood sugar levels remain under better control without the high spikes and dips, you will actually begin to experience more energy. This is because your body is working more efficiently and using its fat stores as fuel. Now you do not have to deal with those post-sugar crashes that often caused you to feel foggy and fatigued. Additionally, your body responds to these positive changes by helping your adrenal glands and thyroid functions to return to healthy levels.

3. Your body will enjoy more nutrients ~ As I have shared before, sugar has absolutely no nutrients in it, yet it is full of calories. When sugar is decreased and slowly eliminated, your body will still need energy and will cause you to experience hunger, but now you will be striving to give it healthy foods for energy. This act alone results in your body receiving more vitamins and valuable nutrients it needs to help you function better. Additionally, the elimination of sugar can also result in weight loss and an improvement in your immune system.

4. Inflammation is reduced ~ Sugar can be referred to as a type of food that causes inflammation. While there are good kinds of inflammation your body goes through to help you fight infections, rebuild muscles after exercising, and to heal wounds, sugar in your system creates too much inflammation. When you create this environment in your body and make it deal with an excess of sugar, it responds by causing inflammatory conditions like arthritis and achiness in your joints, gives yeast (candida) in your body some extra food to thrive on, affects your immune system in a negative way, and even offers food for cancer cells. Simply reducing and eliminating sugar from your body can offer some very positive results by decreasing inflammatory symptoms and may even cause some of them to disappear.

5. Healthier skin ~ Many have no idea how sugar actually damages the collagen in their skin. Collagen is a protein found in our bodies that is like a type of "glue" that holds our tissue together. It accounts for almost one-third of all the protein content in our bodies. It is so prevalent in our bodies that it can be found in our muscles, bones, eyes, intestines, and in the fibrous tissues that exist in our skin. Since sugar is known to damage collagen, its side effects can range from skin that is not very elastic, causing wrinkles at an early age—meaning more than you might otherwise get if you did not consume much sugar. Additionally, eczema and acne can find improvement when sugar is eliminated or drastically reduced.

6. Your sleeping will improve ~ Your body was designed to burn fat throughout the night because fat burns slowly in our bodies and for a long time. Remember, when sugar is elevated in our bloodstream, our bodies use the sugar for fuel instead of fat. When you have sugar in your bloodstream at bedtime, your body will burn this fuel quickly, resulting in a drop in your blood sugar levels. While there is a host of medical explanations on how this works, the result is the wrong kind of fuel for sleeping that causes disruptions in your sleep patterns. This in turn leads to messing up your sleep and appetite hormones, which then affect your ability to feel rested. Consequently, your body quits functioning properly and often causes you to gain weight. Part of the answer is learning to avoid sugary foods and to establish better sleep patterns. Once sugar is greatly reduced, you will begin to notice better sleep, more energy, and possibly even some weight loss.

There are certainly other symptoms that will improve and often disappear as sugar begins to disappear from your body like experiencing less gas, having fewer cravings, and even better mental clarity, but I think you get the idea. Choosing to reduce and even eliminate most sugars, especially added sugars, from your diet means you have everything to gain—except weight!

Chapter 13 - How Can I Handle Sugar Cravings During and After a Detox?

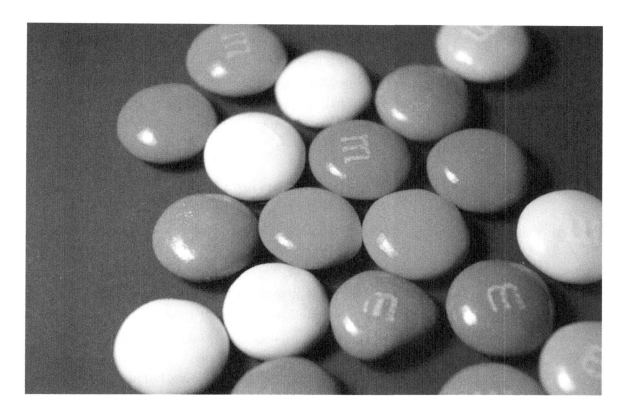

I wish I could tell you that once you are successful with a sugar detox program that you will never have to worry about cravings again, but alas, that would be a lie. As I have shared, sugar is a powerful "drug," and one that we are constantly surrounded with in our daily lives. For these two reasons alone, you invariably will find times when you feel like sugar is hard to resist, especially when something sweet is offered to you. Sometimes you are going to want to eat something sweet because a certain emotion is evoked within you that reminds you of your childhood or a special memory.

To be able to handle moments when you feel tempted to eat sugar, you have to have a plan of action in place—one that you have decided ahead of time to execute when you know temptations will come. Below I have listed a few ideas to help you get through these moments—for those times when you really want to win out over sugar.

However, before I start listing ideas, realize there will be times when you are not feeling out of control or like you cannot be around sugary foods. Sometimes you will choose to enjoy it for the moment, knowing this food is only a temporary pleasure. This is perfectly fine and is not to be viewed as being weak, backsliding or wimping out. Sugar has been with us for a long time and I suspect, will remain with us throughout our lifetime. An occasional indulgence is perfectly fine. Yet, having a lifestyle plan in place on how to handle sugar so you can go back to it will serve you well for times when you may not want to indulge, but you are feeling weak and afraid you might lose control.

One other important point to say here: You have to learn how to tell the difference between hunger and a craving. "Hunger ~ a feeling of discomfort or weakness due to a lack of food, coupled with a need to eat; a compelling need for food." "Craving ~ a powerful desire for something; to long for something; want greatly; desire eagerly."

Do you see the difference between the two? True hunger means you need to eat something. It is almost as if your body has no choice but to consume something to keep functioning. However, a craving is NOT a need! Instead, it is eating that is optional! It does not have to happen in order for your body to function. Cravings offer us choices in how we satisfy them, and how we handle them is critical for learning how to overcome them.

Ideas for Conquering Cravings (During a Detox and for Life)

Whenever you sense a craving for sugar coming over you, try one or more of the following suggestions:

1. Look for a distraction. Because many have grown up with emotional issues related to food (particularly sweets), making a decision to do something else to distract your desire for food could work fabulously. When you feel a craving coming on, change what you are doing. Instead of staying in the house, go for a walk, call a special friend, or get involved in a project. This step may take some time for you to realize what is happening and to find solutions that are effective, but just be aware that this is one way to fight back when an urge for sweets hits you.

2. Drink some water or a refreshing beverage like herbal tea. Cravings sometimes hit us because we are bored, tired, or hungry. A great way to fight off a craving because you think you are hungry is to fill up your stomach with a healthy beverage. Sometimes this in itself is enough to tell your brain that your stomach is full so it can turn off the signal for food and leave you alone.

3. Have a healthy snack readily available. Because sugar cravings can hit you when your blood sugar levels get too low, be ready to fight back with healthy snacks. Keep your home, your purse, and even your desk drawer at work equipped with healthy, sugar free snacks. Stock your refrigerator with carrot chips, salsa, celery, nut butters, beef jerky, cheese sticks, and dill pickles for times when you just have to have something to eat.

4. Grab some protein. Sometimes it may be difficult for you to know if you are experiencing a craving or if you are really hungry. The best way to handle this is to eat some protein. If you are hungry, eating protein supplies valuable nourishment for your body and will satisfy your hungry. However, if it is a craving, eating some protein will often make any previous cravings disappear as well.

5. Satisfy a craving with some fruit and sweet vegetables. While fruits have sweetness, they have a bunch of healthy nutrients to offer your body that sweets such as candy and cakes cannot. Fruit offers you vitamins, minerals, enzymes, and even fiber, which helps to balance out the sugar content in the fruit. In addition, sweet vegetables like carrots, beets, and sweet potatoes—all of which are healthy alternatives to sugary snacks—are helpful in stabilizing your blood sugar levels. In so doing, this will eliminate your cravings, too.

6. Sometimes giving in a little is all you need. While your goal is to eliminate or drastically reduce sugar in your diet, sometimes giving yourself permission to enjoy a little bit of something sweet is fine. It will help you feel like you are not being deprived. The longer you eliminate sugar from your diet, you may discover that even a little sugar seems like a lot.

7. My best tip of all: Eat on a regular basis. Cravings often occur, although not exclusively, because you waited too long between meals to eat something healthy. When your sugar levels drop, that is when cravings are most likely to occur. For most, eating something healthy every 3 to 4 hours keeps cravings away and maintains a nice and stable blood sugar level.

Realize, temptations and cravings are here to stay, but that does not mean that you cannot be prepared. Knowing some things to do, like what I have listed above, will equip you and empower you the next time you are faced with having to choose between giving in to a craving or fighting back.

Chapter 14 – How Can I Eat Out Successfully?

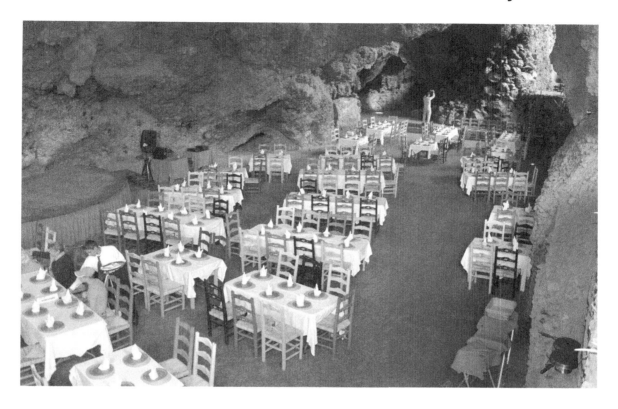

Eating out when you are detoxing will be more difficult to do than staying at home to eat because you know what is in your food when you fix it. Eating out requires a little more work but certainly is not impossible to do. Personally, I almost never eat at a fast-food restaurant because now I know too much of what is healthy to do. I make much of what I eat at home, but when I do go out to eat, I pick restaurants where I know they offer healthy protein dishes without a lot of sauces and additives, along with healthy side dishes consisting of foods that are steamed and grilled and offer healthy salads.

Doing your homework as I have done and putting a workable plan in place will equip you to handle eating out effectively and nutritiously. Here are some tactics you can employ for your next dining experience:

- First things first—Make sure you are dining out because you are hungry. If you are invited out to eat with friends, calmly decide if you are hungry and then order accordingly. If you are not very hungry but you know it will be time to eat soon, order something light like a bowl of vegetable soup and a salad

- Tell the server not to bring bread to the table. Why put yourself through this temptation? Just have your server leave the bread in the kitchen

- Know something about the restaurant where you will be dining. Many restaurants have their menus online so if you know where you will be eating, you can make your decisions rationally ahead of time—before you are hungry

- Focus on ordering a healthy protein first and then decide on the vegetables

- Order baked, broiled and grilled items instead of fried ones

- Order water or herbal tea for your beverage instead of sodas and sugary drinks

- Take your time eating your food. Enjoy it. Savor each bite. Quit when you are full. Take home the leftovers to enjoy for another meal

- If your meal comes with two side items--steamed vegetables and rice, or pasta--ask your server to give you a double order of vegetables instead of a starchy side item. (I do this a lot)

- If you will be dining at a friend's home, ask if you can bring something that will also fit in with your present eating habits

More and more restaurants are catering to the desires of their customers, so decide what you want to eat and order it "your way."

Chapter 15 – What Should My Eating Habits Look Like After I Finish a Detox?

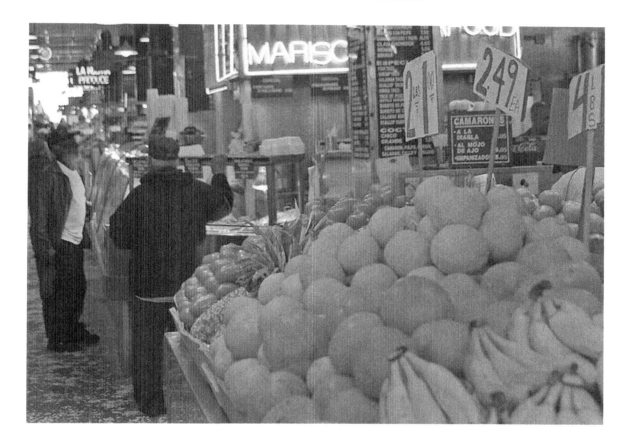

Something I hope that happens for you after your detox is that you choose NOT to return to your previous eating patterns. Having done numerous sugar detoxes myself, I know that each time I conquer one, I find that I am less and less tempted to return to my previous eating habits of consuming sugar. For me, it is now easy to say no to a piece of cake and to walk by a plate of cookies without eating any—something I never thought I would be able to do years ago.

Also, be sure to praise and even reward yourself for what you have accomplished. Whether or not you made it completely through the detox without a slip-up is not what to focus on. Instead, celebrate! You made a decision to take better care of yourself and now you are more aware of the effects of sugar on your body and some things you can do to change the status quo.

Hopefully, you have discovered new ways to eat healthier and now desire to continue doing them for life. I know for me, a few years ago after I did a sugar detox for 30 days, I had no desire to eat bread once it was over. In fact, when I go to a restaurant that features grass-fed hamburgers, I always order mine without the bun. I do not miss it and because I know more about grains, inflammation, etc., I really have no desire to eat them. I will admit this did not happen to me the first time I did a detox, though. This only happened after I had been on a journey of trying different kinds of detox programs before I arrived at this point.

After you complete a sugar detox, you will have some decisions to make. Here are a few things to consider going forward:

1. Take some quiet time to evaluate what you have just been through, and ask yourself some questions. What were some of the hardest foods I had to avoid and not eat while I was detoxing? Now that it is over, do I really want to go back to eating them? Did I discover some new favorite foods? What am I willing to keep doing? What am I not willing to continue doing? Did my family benefit from my detox? How has my detox made me feel (successful, empowered, defeated, healthier)?

2. Investigate how to cook with other forms of sugar. White sugar should now be at the top of your list of foods to avoid; however, think of all the foods and recipes that incorporate it into their finished products. Find out about baking with other sugars like raw honey, pure maple syrup and coconut sugar. While these are still sugars, they are healthier options that bring texture and sweetness to foods you cook.

3. Look at other types of diets. Through my journey of trying different types of detoxes, I have started eating more of a Paleo diet because it focuses on eliminating sugars, grains, and processed foods while concentrating on healthy proteins and fats. Do your own research. Talk to friends you trust. Check out the diet and health section at your local bookstore. Learning what options are available to you can help you with your next steps toward health—and your next detox. <smile>

4. With your awareness for foods elevated, consider how to make lifelong commitments of what you choose to eat:

   - Consult your food journal and look at the sweet things you wrote down that you like to eat. Consider removing one of these sweet foods from your diet each week. Try cutting back on the sugar you put in your tea or do not eat desserts with your dinners for a fixed amount of time

   - Switch to Greek-style yogurt instead of fruit-flavored ones

   - Eat sweet potato fries instead of white potato fries

   - Make your own sauces and dressings instead of buying bottled ones

   - Give up cereal for breakfast. Instead, make healthy frittatas or have a burger with salsa

   - Look for full-fat dairy products instead of low-fat ones that have added sugars

- Use healthy oils in your cooking like coconut, extra virgin olive, and others

- Investigate ways to make your favorite foods without using high carb grains. (This one will keep you busy for awhile)

- Do not be afraid to dine out in restaurants. Instead, investigate different ones and make healthy choices

5. Continue planning healthy meals and snacks. First, focus on having good proteins in your meals and snacks, and have a healthy supply of fats like nuts, nut butters, oils, and butter. Then move on to including vegetables in your meals and snacks. As you know now, being prepared is a huge part of being successful with eating and feeling well

6. Get your family involved. Share with them your health concerns about how you eat as a family and what changes you would like to see happen. Often their input will cause them to take ownership in what you are trying to accomplish which can make transitions easier and more effective

7. Enlist the help of a friend that you trust and who is on the same journey. Spend time with each other and talk on a regular basis. Share ideas and recipes. Be honest about your struggles and victories.

As you can see, many things are affected when you go through a sugar detox—some as soon as you finish and others that will take time to process and implement.

Chapter 16 – Conclusion

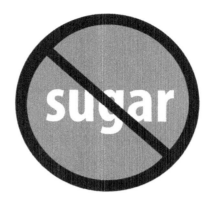

I want to close with a few thoughts concerning your willingness to conduct a sugar detox. First of all, expect it to be difficult; however, expect that you can do it!

While processing the information I have presented here, I hope you have come to see that doing a sugar detox could greatly benefit you and is worth the effort. In doing so, keep the following points in mind:

1. Remember that overcoming the powerful effects that sugar can have on your body, and being able to withdraw from sugar is usually not an issue of willpower—it is more about the biochemical makeup of your body when you begin. Because sugar has been compared to having some of the same effects on your body as cocaine does, you begin to understand that a lot is going on when sugar is in your system. The way your health is affected by the highs and lows of your blood sugar levels, the effects it has on your brains, and the state of your health are all contributing factors that play into your detox.

2. Depending upon the state of your health and how much sugar you are used to ingesting before you start a detox program, you may have to try several times before you are successful all the way through. Realize, this is totally fine! Anytime you are able to get through even one day of a sugar detox program means you have done your body a favor. For many, it requires doing a sugar detox several times before they are able to finish the program. Just remember to celebrate every little victory when you are trying to detox. Besides, if it were easy, you wouldn't need to be reading this book.

3. Depending upon your lifestyle, what you normally eat, and several other factors, I would suggest you do a three-day program your first time or two. You can schedule it over the course of a long weekend and you know that it will be over when you head back to work.

4. Detoxing sugar from your body is a process—one that requires education, willingness, and patience. As you go through a detox, pay attention to the foods you are eating and how your body is reacting. Write in your journal and pay attention to things you believe you could adapt for the rest of your life. Decide what you are willing to do, and not do, and then do them. For a very long time, I routinely enjoyed two pieces of homemade bread with butter for breakfast and a cup of coffee with Splenda®, creamer and some orange juice along with it. Can you even count how many carbohydrates a breakfast like this has? Yet now, I can drink my coffee black whenever I want to, I do not use artificial sweeteners in it, I have not had bread in several years, but I still do have some orange juice every day or two—but only about 8-10 ounces. Orange juice is just something I know I am not going to quit drinking and I am okay with that.

5. Keep researching to learn about ways to handle cravings with sugar. I have read that drinking herbal teas can help; adding cinnamon to a smoothie can help regulate blood sugar; taking supplements like L-glutamine to improve intestinal function and magnesium can help your body with energy production.

With each detox, you will learn something new—about the program and about yourself. And with each one, you will find your limits and experience victories. To be sure, going through a sugar detox has its moments of trials and testing, but each day that you get through with less sugar in your system, the better your health can be.

Chapter 17 – Recipes to Help You Continue to Succeed

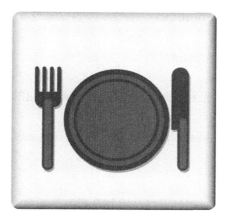

I wanted to end my book by offering you some recipes to help you with your efforts to dramatically reduce sugar in your life.

Breakfast Ideas

Learning to eat differently at breakfast, without the sugary cereals and pastries, offers exciting flavors and nutritious dishes to try. Whether you enjoy a delicious smoothie before leaving the house or you take the time to make a tasty frittata, breakfast offers many new possibilities for you.

Be sure to experiment and try new things.

Here are a few to help get your motor running in the mornings to help you last until lunchtime.

Raspberry Smoothie

Ingredients:

- 1½ cups nut milk (coconut or almond)

- 1 small handful arugula

- 1 small handful baby spinach

- 4 strawberries, frozen

- 1 cup fresh raspberries, frozen

- ½ teaspoon pure vanilla extract

- 1 scoop protein powder (optional. If you use this, be sure to find one with very little sugar)

Directions:

1. In your blender, pour in the nut milk

2. Now put in the arugula and spinach

3. Place the frozen berries on next and then pour in your vanilla

4. Process on high until you achieve your desired consistency. You may need to add a little more milk if it is too thick

Makes 1 large serving or 2 smaller ones

Quiche Cups

When you are trying to keep the sugar content down in the foods you eat, eliminating grains can help a lot but can be a challenge to figure out what to eat for breakfast.

This recipe is one that I have enjoyed making for my family. Not only are they easy, but they are a fun presentation, too. Consider making more than you need for one meal and keep them in the refrigerator. They are easy to reheat and are great for when you need something nutritious when you are in a hurry.

Ingredients:

- 2 tablespoons coconut oil

- ½ pound of meat (ground pork or turkey works well)

- 1 small onion, peeled and chopped

- 1 bell pepper, seeded and diced

- ½ cup fresh sliced mushrooms

- ¼ cup fresh salsa

- 6 eggs

- ⅓ cup shredded aged cheddar cheese or Parmesan

- ¾ cup almond or coconut milk

Directions:

1. Begin by preheating your oven to 325 degrees F

2. Grease a muffin tin using coconut oil or coconut spray

3. In a large frying pan on your stovetop, put in the coconut oil in to heat it up

4. Place your meat into the heated coconut oil and brown

5. Now, drain the meat by placing it on a paper towel or strain it and set aside

6. Now return to your frying pan on the stovetop and add a little more coconut oil if necessary

7. Once heated, place the onion, bell pepper, and mushrooms

8. Season as you like and cook until these are tender

9. Now add the fresh salsa and cook until most of the liquid is reduced

10. In a medium mixing bowl, add the eggs and beat until blended

11. Add the cheese and nut milk and blend together

12. Place the meat into the egg mixture along with the vegetables from the frying pan when they are fully cooked

13. Mix thoroughly

14. Now evenly divide the meat/egg mixture into your muffin cups

15. Place the muffin tin into your preheated oven and bake for 20-25 minutes. Make sure they are fully cooked in the middle and are a nice golden brown color on top

16. Allow them to cool for a few minutes, then remove from the muffin tin and enjoy

Makes about 12 muffins

Blackberry Bars

If you try to eliminate regular grains from your cooking, you will find that almond flour and coconut flour offer you some nice alternatives. This recipe also contains some raw honey which will add sugar to your recipe so you may want to try it with less or none at all. Try this recipe and see what you think.

Ingredients:

- ½ cup unsweetened shredded coconut

- 1 cup almond flour

- 1 teaspoon cinnamon

- ½ teaspoon baking soda

- 1 teaspoon baking powder

- ½ teaspoon sea salt

- ¼ cup raw honey

- 2 ripe bananas, mashed

- 2 eggs

- 1 teaspoon pure vanilla extract

- ¾ cup almond or coconut milk (1/2 + a little extra)

- 2 tablespoons coconut oil (melted but not hot)

- 1 cup blackberries, fresh or thawed

Directions:

1. Preheating your oven to 350 degrees F

2. In an 8 x 8 inch baking dish, grease the bottom and sides with coconut oil

3. Using a large mixing bowl, place the coconut, almond flour, cinnamon, baking soda, baking powder, and salt and mix thoroughly to combine

4. In a separate bowl, mash your banana

5. Now stir in the eggs, vanilla, ½ cup of the nut milk, and the oil

6. Stir vigorously to combine thoroughly

7. Pour the wet ingredients into the dry ingredients and mix until all ingredients are moist

8. Fold in the blackberries

9. You want your batter to be kind of like a cookie batter. Feel free to add extra milk if it is too thick

10. Add your mashed bananas, eggs, oil, vanilla, and only 1/4 cup of the nut milk

11. Pour batter into your prepared baking dish and place it in the oven

12. Bake it for approximately 40 minutes. It is done when the sides begin to come away from the sides of the pan and it is a golden brown color

13. Once it is finished cooking, allow it to stay in the pan until completely cooled

14. Slice and enjoy

Lunch Ideas

If you work outside the home or attend school, lunches can be a challenge when you are trying to keep sugar to a minimum. Planning ahead helps tremendously with lunches. You can fix them the night before or early in the morning before you leave (if you have enough time). Put your food into a thermos and insulated container and you are ready for your next hunger attack.

Sweet Potato Soup

Ingredients:

- 1 tablespoon coconut oil

- 1 tablespoon coconut flour

- 1½ cups chicken stock

- ¼ teaspoon ground ginger (or fresh, to taste)

- ⅛ teaspoon ground nutmeg

- ⅛ teaspoon ground cinnamon

- Salt and pepper to taste

- 1 cup coconut milk

- 1 large sweet potato, cooked, peeled and cubed

Directions:

1. On your stovetop, use a medium-sized pot and combine the oil and flour until blended

2. Turn the flame up to medium and continually stir the oil and flour until it becomes a golden brown color. You want it to resemble the color of caramel

3. Now add in the stock and bring the liquid to a boil

4. When a boil occurs, turn the flame down to a low setting and add in your spices and coconut milk

5. Stir thoroughly, then gently add in the potato cubes

6. Cook for 10 minutes

7. Now carefully add the mixture to your blender or use an immersion blender stick to create a smooth consistency

8. Serve and enjoy or pack it for a portable lunch

Makes 3 - 4 servings

Fruit Salad with Chicken

Fruit salad with chicken will supply you with good sugars and a healthy protein to get you through the toughest of days. This salad should keep you satisfied until dinnertime arrives.

Ingredients:

- ¼ cup chopped red onion

- 2 celery stalks, finely chopped

- ¼ cup chopped pecans (optional)

- ½ cup dried unsweetened cranberries

- 1 (12 ounce) can of white chicken

- ¼ cup mayonnaise

Directions:

1. In a medium-sized bowl, add the onion, celery, pecans, and cranberries and stir to mix

2. Break up the chicken into small pieces, then add to the bowl

3. Add in the mayonnaise and mix thoroughly

4. This salad makes a great sandwich when you wrap it inside of large lettuce leaves. It can also be used as a dip for enjoying apple slices, celery stick and carrot chips

Makes 2 - 3 servings

Lettuce Wraps

This sandwich filling is packed with goodness. With avocado, chicken, and the refreshing taste of cilantro and lime, it will cause your mouth to explode with wonderful flavors.

Ingredients:

- 1 avocado

- 2 tomatoes, chopped

- ½ bell pepper, chopped

- 1 chicken breast, cooked and cubed

- 1 clove garlic, minced

- ¼ onion, chopped

- Juice from 1 lime

- 4 big lettuce leaves

- 1 sprig fresh cilantro, minced

Directions:

1. In a medium-sized bowl, mash up the avocado until you have a nice, smooth consistency

2. Stir in the tomatoes, bell pepper, chicken, garlic, onion, and lime

3. Spread out evenly between your lettuce leaves, then sprinkle on the fresh cilantro

4. Roll the lettuce leaf up like a burrito and enjoy

Makes 4 servings

Dinner Ideas

Vegetable Stew with Hamburger

This is one of my favorite soups to make, especially when there will be numerous people eating. My family always enjoys it and I make sure there is enough for leftovers for lunches and another round for dinner. It also freezes really well. It tastes great coming out of a crockpot, but it can also be made on your stovetop in a big Dutch oven if you do not have time to prepare it early in the day. Just make sure you allow enough time for the carrots to soften.

Ingredients:

- 2 tablespoons olive oil

- 2 pounds lean ground beef

- 4 stalks celery, stalks

- 2 onions, chopped

- 2 cups fresh mushrooms

- 2 bell pepper – any color – seeded and chopped

- 2 quarts beef broth

- 4 cups fresh green beans, snapped into bite-sized pieces, or the equivalent of frozen or canned

- 5 carrots peeled and sliced

- 2 (15 ounce) cans tomato sauce

- 2 teaspoons celery seed

- 1 tablespoon kosher or sea salt

- 2 teaspoons coarse black pepper

Directions:

1. First, plug in your crockpot and turn it up to HIGH while you are preparing your ingredients

2. On your stovetop in a frying pan, brown your ground beef

3. Drain if necessary, then place in your crockpot

4. Return to your pan on the stovetop and add in the celery, onions, mushrooms, and bell peppers and cook until tender

5. Now add the vegetables to your crockpot

6. Pour in the broth, green beans, carrots and tomato sauce and stir to mix

7. Finally, add the celery seed, salt and pepper and stir

8. Put the lid on your crockpot and turn the temperature down to LOW

9. Cook for 7 to 8 hours, making sure the carrots are soft

Makes 8-10 servings

Chicken Cacciatore

Chicken Cacciatore is delicious and not difficult to make. While this recipe is written to be made in a crockpot, it can also be prepared on your stovetop.

Something I have started doing all the time with this recipe is I now serve it over spaghetti squash. It acts just like pasta but is so much healthier.

Ingredients:

- 2 bell peppers, seeded and chopped

- 8 ounce package of fresh mushrooms

- 4 garlic cloves, minced

- 2 onions, peeled and chopped

- 6 boneless, skinless chicken breasts

- ¾ cup white cooking wine

- ¼ cup tomato paste

- 14.5 ounce can diced tomatoes, undrained

- 1½ cups chicken stock

- 3 bay leaves

- 2 teaspoons Italian seasoning

- 1 teaspoon salt

- 1 teaspoon pepper

- ¼ cup water

- 2 tablespoons arrowroot powder

Directions:

1. As you are getting your ingredients ready, turn on your crockpot to HIGH

2. To the bottom of your crockpot, place the bell peppers, mushrooms, garlic and onions

3. Now place the chicken breasts on top of the vegetables

4. In a medium-sized bowl, combine the cooking wine, tomato paste, tomatoes with the juice, and the chicken stock and blend

5. Add this liquid to your crockpot

6. Place the bay leaves, Italian seasoning, salt, and pepper on top of the ingredients

7. Place the cover on the crockpot and turn it down to LOW

8. Cook on LOW for 7 to 8 hours (or you can leave it on HIGH and cook for 3 to 4 hours)

9. After the allotted time, remove the pieces of chicken breast and place in a bowl where you can shred the pieces

10. While the chicken is out of the crockpot, take a small bowl and mix the water and arrowroot powder together until it is smooth

11. Add the arrowroot liquid to the liquid in your crockpot and mix. This will thicken your sauce

12. Now mix in the shredded chicken with the sauce, replace the cover and allow the sauce to heat back up for approximately 30 more minutes to achieve its final thickening

13. It is now ready to be enjoyed

Makes 8 servings

Pizza without a Crust

This pizza can be made without cheese if dairy is a problem for you or someone in your family. However, if you enjoy cheese as I do, you will find this crust-less pizza a winner—and without as many carbs as regular pizza.

Ingredients:

- ¼ cup aged Parmesan cheese (optional)

- 2 pounds ground beef

- 2 garlic cloves, finely chopped

- 2 teaspoons dried oregano

- ½ teaspoon dried onion powder

- 2 teaspoons sea salt

- 2 eggs

- ½ cup of 100% tomato sauce

- 1 tablespoon Italian seasoning

- ½ bell pepper, chopped

- Pitted black olives, sliced

- 6 to 8 fresh mushrooms, sliced

- Finely chopped cooked meat as a topping for your pizza

- 1 red onion, thinly sliced

- 8 ounces aged cheddar cheese, shredded (optional)

Directions:

1. Preheat your oven to 450 degrees F

2. Using a cookie sheet with a small lip around it, lightly grease it with coconut oil

3. In a medium-sized bowl, add the cheese, ground beef, garlic, oregano, onion powder, and salt

4. Break the eggs into the bowl and thoroughly combine all the ingredients until the consistence is the same throughout

5. Dump the mixture out onto the cookie sheet and press it out with your hands to make the "crust."

6. Place in your preheated oven and cook for 12 to 15 minutes to make sure your crust is cooked through

7. Remove the cookie sheet from the oven and place on your countertop

8. Return to your oven and turn it to broil

9. Spread the tomato sauce over the top of your crust

10. Sprinkle on the Italian seasoning

11. Now spread the bell pepper, olives, mushrooms, chopped meat, and onions over the crust, followed by the cheese

12. Place the cookie sheet under your broiler and allow the ingredients to get hot and the cheese to brown—approximately 6 to 8 minutes

13. Remove your pizza from under the broiler, allow it to cool slightly, then slice and eat

Dessert Ideas

If you are up for the challenge, I have a few recipes for you that do not contain grains, which are high in carbs. Instead, they are made with nuts, almond flour and coconut flour. These ingredients are not as difficult to find now as they once were, especially because many of the larger grocery chains are carrying them now in their stores.

While there are some natural sweeteners in the recipes, these are to be enjoyed on occasion—not every day or night. Plus, you can cut back on the amounts if you wish.

Lemon Bars

Ingredients:

Topping

- 1 cup fresh lemon juice (about 8 lemons)

- ½ cup raw honey

- 6 eggs

- ½ cup coconut oil

Crust

- 1 cup macadamia nuts

- 1 cup raw almonds

- 2 eggs

- ½ cup coconut oil, melted

- ¼ cup raw honey

- Unsweetened shredded coconut for topping

Directions:

1. Preheat your oven to 400 degrees F

2. Lightly grease a rectangular baking dish with coconut oil along the bottom and sides

3. On your stovetop, using a medium-sized pan, place the lemon juice, honey, and eggs and stir

4. Add in the coconut oil next

5. Using a medium heat setting, stir this mixture until it comes to a boil and thickens

6. Take it off the heat

7. Now pour the egg mixture into a bowl and allow it to cool completely in your refrigerator

8. While it is cooling, take your food processor and put in the macadamias and almonds and pulse to create small chunks. (Do not process too long or you will end up with flour)

9. Now pour the chunky nut mixture into a medium-sized bowl and add the eggs, coconut oil and honey and stir thoroughly

10. Spread out this mixture evenly in your dish

11. Place it in the oven and bake it for approximately 20 minutes. The crust should turn a light golden brown when it is done

12. Take it out of the oven and allow it to cool completely

13. Once cooled, take your lemon mixture out of the refrigerator and spread it out evenly over your crust

14. Now sprinkle the shredded coconut over the lemon mixture

15. Place a cover or plastic wrap over the dish and return it to your refrigerator to cool and set up

Pumpkin Pie

Ingredients:

Crust:

- ¼ cup coconut oil, melted
- 2 teaspoons pure maple syrup
- 3 egg whites
- ¼ teaspoon sea salt
- ½ cup coconut flour
- ½ cup unsweetened coconut flakes

Filling:

- 3 whole eggs
- ¾ cup full fat coconut milk
- 1 teaspoon pure vanilla extract
- 1/8 cup pure maple syrup
- 1 tablespoon pumpkin pie spice
- 1½ cups 100% pumpkin puree
- ½ teaspoon sea salt

Directions:

1. Preheat your oven to 400 degrees F
2. Using a 9-inch pie pan, grease the bottom and sides with coconut oil
3. Pour the coconut oil, maple syrup, egg whites, salt, coconut flour, and coconut flakes into a medium-sized bowl
4. Using a hand mixer, mix to thoroughly blend the ingredients and make sure there are no lumps

5. Pour this mixture into your pie pan, using your hands or the bottom of a measuring cup or glass to pack it firmly and evenly across the bottom

6. Cook the crust for approximately 10 minutes. It should be slightly browned

7. Now LOWER the temperature of your oven by turning it down to 350 degrees F

8. Using the same bowl you used for the crust, place the eggs in the bowl and process on high for 2 minutes to allow the eggs to increase in size

9. Now add in all the remaining ingredients

10. Once again, use your hand mixer and blend the mixture on high for 2 more minutes

11. Now pour this mixture into your crust

12. Return the pie pan to your oven and cook for approximately 35 minutes. Make sure the center is firm and not wiggly in the middle

13. Let your pie cool completely and then cut and serve

Makes one 9-inch pie

Raspberry Cake in a Mug

Here is a delicious dessert you can make anytime you want a treat. You can either microwave it for a few minutes or take the time to cook it in the oven. I happen to like the finished product better when it comes out of the oven.

The directions are for one serving but you can have family and friends make one of their own—just the way they like them—cook them all at once in the oven, and enjoy them together.

Ingredients:

- 8 fresh raspberries

- 2-inch slice of banana (the riper, the sweeter)

- 1 teaspoon pure vanilla extract

- 2 teaspoons raw honey

- 1 egg

- ½ teaspoon baking powder

- 1/8 teaspoon sea salt

- 1½ tablespoons coconut flour

Directions:

1. Decide if you are going to bake your mug cake or cook it in the microwave

2. If cooking it in the oven, then preheat your oven to 350 degrees F

3. Take a large mug or a ramekin, place the raspberries and banana slice in the bottom

4. Use and fork and mash them up together and blend

5. On top of the fruit, add the vanilla, honey, and egg

6. Mix vigorously to blend it all together

7. Now add in the baking powder, salt, and flour

8. Mix vigorously again so you do not end up with lumpy flour or spots where the baking powder did not blend in with the other ingredients

9. Place your container on a baking sheet and place it in your preheated oven

10. Bake for 30 minutes

11. Allow the cake to cool and make sure you handle the container carefully

If using a microwave: Put your ramekin or mug in your microwave and cook it on high for approximately 2 to 2½ minutes

Makes 1 serving

Free Download of Recipes

As you did with the grocery list offered earlier in this book, just go to http://tenfingerspublishing.com/sugar-detox-recipes/ where you can download a PDF and print it out to use them at home.

Hopefully, these recipes will equip and empower you as you attempt to make positive changes in your life to decrease your intake of sugars as it helps you and those you love live healthier lives. Enjoy!

Chapter 18 – Some Additional Resources

Below are some resources you may want to consult as you continue to work toward keeping sugars out of your diet. Many I have read and have personal experience with while others are ones I know about from sources I trust.

1. The 21-Day Sugar Detox by Diane Sanfilippo ~ http://www.the21daysugardetox.com

2. The Whole30® Program by Dallas & Melissa Hartwig ~ http://www.whole9life.com/2013/08/the-whole30-program/

(Their book, **It Starts with Food** is an excellent read for conducting a sugar detox, too. It goes hand-in-hand with their Whole30® Program)

3. Mommy Run Fast ~ 7 day detox programs that start about once every month ~ http://www.mommyrunfast.com/sugar-detox/

There are many diets and ways of eating to choose from. One that advocates eliminating sugar is the Paleo Diet®. It focuses on grass-fed meats and dairy, no grains (high in carbs), wholesome vegetables, nuts and seeds, and little to no processing of foods. I have watched as this area has exploded with new books and cookbooks coming into the marketplace. If you are interested in trying to keep sugars out of your diet after you have finished your detox, you may want to consider looking into this lifestyle.

Here are a few I have purchased and read:

1. Mark Sisson's books. Be sure to check out his website at: http://www.MarksDailyApple.com

2. Books by Rob Wolf. His website can be found at: http://www.RobbWolf.com

3. Sarah Fragoso's website and books: http://www.EverydayPaleo.com

4. The Foodee: http://www.thefoodee.com/

5. For information that is easy to read with practical information to get started quickly:

- **Going Paleo: A Quick Start Guide to a Gluten-Free Diet** by Amelia Simons (She also has a line of cookbooks you could enjoy as I have. The easiest way to find them is to go to her author page on Amazon: http://www.amazon.com/author/ameliasimons

6. Danielle Walker's website and new book called, **Against All Grain**: http://www.againstallgrain.com/

There are certainly many more but these should help get you started. Enjoy your research!

About the Author

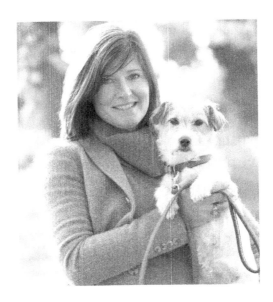

Like many of us, Charlotte remembers a childhood of being described as "chubby," and college years of experimenting with "every diet known to man," had very little effect. Even classes on nutrition yielded minimal results.

Finally, as a married woman, Charlotte was able to surround herself with friends who lovingly supported her and gave her the encouragement and information she needed to understand how her body worked. It was then she was able to begin to see positive changes.

Through extensive research and conducting her own interviews with medical professionals and people who had lost weight, she changed her eating habits, eliminated most sugars from her diet, and became active in sports—something she was never able to do as a child.

Charlotte now enjoys teaching others about health, exercise, and healthy cooking—through her writing, and through cooking classes held in her home.

CPSIA information can be obtained at www.ICGtesting.com
Printed in the USA
LVOW02s0941110114

369015LV00007BA/69/P